Expert Appraisals of the Book

The 'Midwife Apprentice' is a smashing book, which is an altogether easy read. I totally recommend this historical memoir to anyone considering a career in midwifery. The stories regaled beautifully capture the art of midwifery through the recall of experiences encountered by a pioneer midwife in Milwaukee, WI, USA. Throughout my grazes on this memoir, I resonated with much of the narrative. During my own 40-year career as a midwife in the UK, there have been aspects of learning the craft, reflections upon birthing experiences, normal straightforward physiological births, spectacular gymnastic birthing feats, episodes that challenge and shape learning, reading required to gain greater depth of understanding, episodes where birth became traumatic, premature labours, and encounters of adjacent medical complications. I observe that childbirth between 1875 and 2023, whether in Scotland or the US, has numerous unanticipated events and happy outcomes. Well done, Susan Fleming, another spectacular book for any woman's shelf.

Prof Caroline J Hollins Martin PhD MPhil BSc RM RGN MBPsS
Senior Fellow HA | Professor in Midwifery
Subject Lead for Midwifery in the School of Health & Social Care
Edinburgh Napier University | Scotland (UK)

The Midwife Apprentice is a true-to-life story of a young girl drawn into midwifery by a compelling desire to help women in their time of need. Alice experiences the beauty of birth, success, disappointment, and deep sorrow as she assists women in difficult conditions and circumstances in labor and delivery. I was totally taken in by the book, an absolute must-read for anyone touched by childbirth.

Margene Chantry, BSN, RN, L & D Nurse
Mother of 18, Washington

The Midwife Apprentice is a fascinating story of a young woman learning the art and science of midwifery in the 1880s in Midwest America, where formal midwifery education was not yet in place. Luckily, Alice had her mother and grandmother as teachers, who were both experienced in midwifery and nursing. Although birthing is hard work and sometimes a harrowing experience, Alice learned that our job as midwives is to support the normal physiologic processes for the best outcomes! As I read the book, my thoughts turned to my own continuous learning from women and families after almost five decades of practice and teaching midwifery. The joys and challenges of being a midwife are brought to life in the book. Alice Ada Wood, a young pioneer midwife, was learning to be attentive, skilled, and caring for the women and families she served. I can hardly wait to read what she does in the future!

Katherine Camacho Carr, PhD, ARNP, CNM, FACNM, FAAN
Professor Emerita, Seattle University College of Nursing
kcarr@seattleu.edu

The Midwife's Apprentice is an enjoyable and realistic look at a fascinating time in history. It sensitively looks at the highs and lows of midwifery and coming of age as a woman in a time when women had little autonomy in decision-making. As a midwife, it reminded me of the struggles and growth during my own time as a new student learning this unique profession and how to be "with women". This book will leave the reader with a desire to serve others without judgment—instead, with love and discernment. Highly recommend!

Sarah Simmons LM
Licensed Midwife | Homebirthing Mother

Susan is an excellent writer with a talent for bringing her characters to life. I found one of her stories particularly enjoyable, where Alice experiences her first hunting trip while being mentored by her father. The story beautifully captures how the experience of hunting goes beyond just the hunt itself. It also allows Alice to bond more closely with her father. The story is set in Wisconsin during the late 1800s when hunting was a common way for people to contribute to their food supply.

Rick Brazell Avid Hunter
President and Founder of First Hunt Foundation

The Midwife Apprentice captivates readers by bringing to life an in-depth account of a young woman's life entering into a challenging role as a mid-1800s midwife. I found the author's blending of her medical experience, extensive research, and colorful personal family history resulted in a fascinating story. I will be looking forward to the next book that follows!

Debe Breckenridge RN IBCLC

This book is a fascinating read for anyone interested in women's health and childbirth stories from America during the late 1800s. The author's insight into maternity care and natural storytelling ability makes this book particularly appealing to those involved or interested in women's health and the history of childbirth.

Denise O'Brien, PhD RM I Assistant Professor/
Associate Dean for Undergraduate Studies I Lecturer in Midwifery
University College of Dublin, Ireland

While reading The Midwife Apprentice, I was frequently reminded of the student midwives I educate today and how, as much as things change in the world, some things stay the same. The process of childbirth was then and is now a normal life event; complications can happen, but for the most part, birth proceeds smoothly when not interfered with. As I educate today's student midwives to practice in the community settings of home and birth centers, it reminds me of the challenges Alice faced in her frontier experiences - those who care for birthing families must be both knowledgeable as well as confident in their skills. What we call the apprenticeship model today was the standard way of learning a trade throughout history. As a midwife approaching her 40th year of caring for birthing families, I'm proud to remember that I began as an apprentice and went on to further my education, much like Alice did. Many of us have midwifery ancestors. They are just unknown to us, which makes these stories all the more precious when they are told. Bravo to Susan Fleming for bringing the stories of her great-grandmother to the written page.

Colleen Donovan-Batson, MS, CNM, ARNP, FACNM
Adjunct Faculty, Midwife Program, Southwest Wisconsin Technical College

Midwife Apprentice
*Alice Ada Wood
Milwaukee Pioneer Midwife
The Early Years*

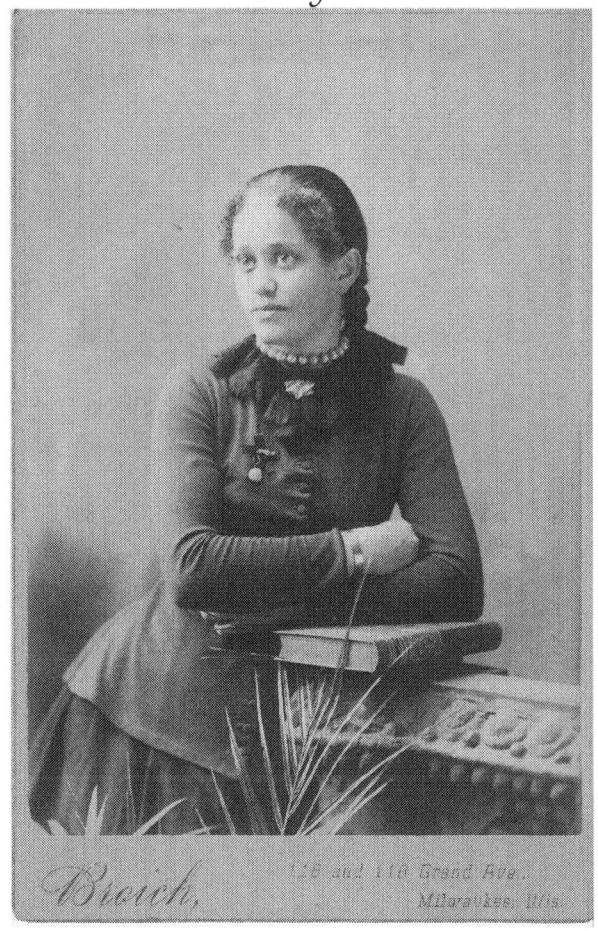

As told by her great-granddaughter
SUSAN E. FLEMING RN PhD
Perinatal Clinical Nurse Special

Alice Ada Wood: Midwife Apprentice

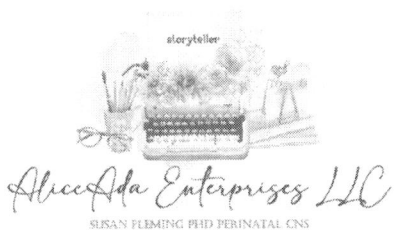

Aliceada Enterprises, LLC
Edition 1 August 1st 2023
Susan E. Fleming PhD, CNS
Perinatal Clinical Nurse Specialist

Editor
Bridgette Tuckfield

Technical Advisors
Edward Oscar Fleming CRNA
Harrison E. Fleming D.O. Internal Medicine

Library of Congress
Published in the United States of America
Copyright © 2023 Susan E. Fleming
All rights reserved.
ISBN: 9798370397622

Alice Ada Wood: Midwife Apprentice

DEDICATION

This book is dedicated to mothers and all who have (or will) compassionately support a woman-with-child to accomplish the incredible feat and miracle of birthing.

I bequeath this book to midwives, nurses, doulas, birth attendants, family members, and birth educators who make birth safe in the homes and hospitals. And to the physicians supporting women during birth, including the womens' choices of where to birth.

Furthermore, may all unclaimed children find a place to call home and people to love them.

I hope that this book can be an example to call on all to see beyond the obvious and take part in discovering and creating the future.

Alice Ada Wood: Midwife Apprentice

Disclaimer: The material in this book is intended to be *informational* and of *historical* interest **only**. It is absolutely not meant to be used as medical advice for actual births.

<u>Certain procedures and treatments used in this book are harmful to mothers and/or their babies.</u>

Please contact a birthing professional during pregnancy and birthing.

Please be aware that the contents of this book may be distressing and could potentially bring up traumatic memories. It is important to approach the material with caution and take breaks as needed while reading.

This book may be used in conjunction with current textbooks as a means to compare and contrast birthing practices today with those from 150 years ago.

Alice Ada Wood: Midwife Apprentice

Author's Notes – Preface

This book serves as a prequel to Seattle Pioneer Midwife and is based on the early years (1880s-1890s) of my great-grandmother Alice Ada Wood and her family in Wisconsin before their westward migration. The storyline takes place during a period when childbirth in uneducated America could be perilous, resulting in tragic outcomes. However, good outcomes prevailed for most births in the American frontier through the wisdom of everyday women who dutifully mentored the next generation. As a young woman, Alice had to navigate through various hindrances as she attended births, such as preeclampsia, breech birth, retained placenta, hemorrhage, and even death. This book is written from Alice's perspective as a young midwife apprentice, delving into her fears, achievements, and traumatic events. Many of the stories in this book are derived from my family stories and personal experiences of birth as a mother, nurse, birthing researcher, or as my time as a midwife apprentice (2017-2018). I was privileged to hear countless women in my life share their coveted birthing stories. I consider the grand multiparous women who birthed five or more babies as birthing experts in the field. I gathered useful advice from skillful nurses, physicians, and mothers during birth. During my time as a midwife apprentice, I was fortunate to be mentored by accomplished midwives who generously shared their valuable guidance and insights. Therefore, I was able to assist many women in achieving normal physiological births, allowing them to respond to their bodies just as women have done for thousands of years.

Reading this book can help readers gain a profound appreciation for midwives' work and challenges. It is a captivating read for anyone interested in midwifery or seeking an engaging book.

Alice Ada Wood: Midwife Apprentice

Table of Contents

1. **Learning the Craft:** *Apprenticing with Maw 1880* — 17
2. **Reflecting on Birthing:** *Processing the Horror and Returning to Normalcy 1880* — 53
3. **Starting a New Year:** *Normal Physiological Birth 1881* — 63
4. **Birthing:** *Acrobatics 1882* — 91
5. **Refining the Craft:** *Not the Head – Then What? 1884* — 113
6. **Educating the Midwest:** *Birthing & Nursing 1885* — 137
7. **Experiencing Violence:** *Sins of the Lawless 1885* — 155
8. **Birthing-too-Soon:** *Multiples, Diseases, or Violence? 1886* — 171
9. **Moving Forward:** *Tricks & Skills of the Trade 1886* — 191
10. **Birthing Science:** *Headaches & Visual Disturbances 1889* — 207
11. **Healing:** *Can a Hunt Bring Me Peace? 1890* — 223
12. **Creating Large Babies:** *Looking Like a Turtle 1890* — 237
13. **Standing with my Love:** *Can He Protect Me? 1891* — 255
14. **Finding Peace:** *Coming Full Circle 1892* — 267

Birthing – Current Definitions & Explanations — 287

Upcoming Releases — 293

Alice Ada Wood: Midwife Apprentice

CHAPTER 1
LEARNING THE CRAFT:
APPRENTICING WITH MAW
1880 - MILWAUKEE

I scaled down the ladder from the loft and entered the gathering room.

"Not much happening," I announced. "It's a quiet night."

Maw looked at me with shame. "Alice, what the heck are you saying, girl?"

Grandma French called out, "Oh, Alice, you just put a curse on this home. Your Maw will now be presented with complicated births all night!"

"Are you kiddin' me? Look at this place," I shot back at my family. "Not much is happening. In fact, not much happening all week. Yeah, Pa should be returning with Eddie from their hunting trip. But that's about it. Maw and Beulah may leave for a birth. But not very exciting for me." I turned to my mother. "Maw, Beu started helping you when she was twelve. Why not me?"

My sister Beulah called out. "Alice, you aren't suited to help Maw. You are too young to go help women birth. You will get scared and won't be much help."

Maw and Grandma nodded their heads in agreement. With a satisfied smile, Beulah left to tend to the animals in the barn.

I shrugged my shoulders and walked away to look out the front window. I gazed at Beu walking up to the barn.

I worried Beulah might be right; assisting women with birth might be more than I could bear. I reckon I may not be ready to attend a birth. But I still desire to attend, as I yearn to help others and contribute to the family. I am twelve years old. I know how babies are born.

Maw, Beu, and Grandma French are always talking about birthing. They speak to each other like I don't understand.

But I do.

Later that evening, my family gathered in the front room after supper. Maw was sitting by the door knitting, Beu was reading her books, and Grandma was sitting in her favorite soft chair beside the crackling fire and reading our family Bible.

Pa and my older brother Eddie entered the house. They were returning from a hunting trip, and we were eager to hear their stories. I especially found Eddie's perspective of the hunt thrilling.

They sat around the table, and we gathered to listen.

Eddie recalled to us, "I did it! I stalked out a buck. Then shot him with my rifle. I hit him just behind the shoulders. He bolted through the forest, but we soon found him dead. Pa says I hit his lungs."

"Yep, he tracked and killed it with a single shot," Pa said, with a smile that I couldn't ever recall seeing for me. I turned my face to the fire as I stoked it to mask any signs of jealousy.

"It's good he didn't blow off his foot with a single shot, a boy that young," Maw bellowed.

Maw wasn't the only lady in the house who thought Eddie was too young to hunt. Grandma and Beu nodded in agreement.

I did not join in. I thought: *Good for you, Eddie.*

The hunters began to unwind as they raised their legs on a table near the couch.

I probed. "Pa, when do I get to go on a hunt?"

"You really want to hunt, don't you, Alice?" Pa answered.

"Of course, I do. It sure beats the humdrum life I have on our small farm out of town," I retorted.

He didn't answer. I looked over to Pa…to see him close his eyes to sleep.

"Doesn't anyone take me seriously in this house?" I complained.

No one answered.

I felt ignored as we settled into our usual routines after the excitement of the hunting stories.

Maw had wandered into the kitchen to make fried apples for a late-night snack. Grandma French moved over to another chair next to the stove. This cozy place allowed her to hear and oversee our family conversations. She pulled out her yarn and started to knit as she watched Maw cooking in an old worn-out frying pan that wobbled as she cooked.

Tonight, the wobbling seemed to set Grandma off. "Somebody needs to buy a suitable frying pan for this house!" she roared, startling us. "I am going to town to pick up a fitting frying pan myself, dang ya!"

Grandma didn't say much, but when she did, we listened.

Pa opened his eyes and countered, "This somebody says our current frying pan is more than suitable!"

Grandma sneered. "The local hardware store in town just got a shipment of frying pans at a reasonable price, you know."

Pa declared, "Grandma French is a know-it-all and a busybody."

I feared those two would kill each other one day.

Suddenly, we heard a thumping knock on the door. We get knocks at all hours, but this one was different. Not the knock, maybe — but certainly the yelling it came along with. Eddie and I ran to the door and peeked out the window next to the door.

An elderly man stood on the doorstep. It was Albert, the man from town who made a living from his horse and carriage service.

He yelled at the top of his lungs between labored breaths. "*Clara*! I need your help! Please come to the door. *Hurry.*"

Maw calmly hollered back from the kitchen while stirring the frying pan. "*No problem*, Albert. I hear ya." Maw took the ladle out of the pan, laid it to the side, and walked unhurriedly to the front door. I am amazed at how she keeps calm when others are distressed.

As she reached him, Albert spoke low and fast. "I'll

wait in the carriage for ya. It's a birth. Just a young girl…real sick with fever. *Hurry!*"

Suddenly, Maw seemed to realize the urgency of this situation. She quickly grabbed her bags by the door, although her face stayed calm. She looked at me with piercing eyes. "Alice, call out for Beulah. She is out at the barn breaking down the haystacks for tomorrow's morning feed."

I didn't want to waste time. So, I ran to the barn as fast as I could.

The full moon lit up the trail. Thankfully, the cool air was crisp and clear, making it easier to see where I was running. But as I got closer to the barn, the ground became wet with cow muck, and it slowed me down. *Yuck!*

Before I reached the barn, Beu came out, supporting her bloody hand. I'd learn later that she had cut her hand badly with a knife she was using to open the haystacks.

I hollered at her. "Maw needs you to attend a birth with her *now!*"

She ran up to the house as fast as she could, wrapping her hand with her apron. I followed her bloody trail close behind as we quickly returned to the house.

When Maw returned from taking her birthing bag to the carriage, she found Beu dripping blood all over the kitchen floor.

Maw gave Beulah a harsh glare. "What did you do to yourself, Beu? You're a bloody mess…and you're not coming with me. I am going to Gertie's house down by the shipyards. That cut-up hand would be left with degradation of the flesh. They are filthy people at that house. Pierson, take care of Beu."

Beulah hung her head as she trudged over to Pa. I felt a bit of sorrow for her as she walks away.

Maw pointed to me. "Alice, you are coming with me!"

"Me?" I asked. Was I hearing this right?

Maw said, "Is there anyone else in this house named Alice?"

"No."

"Get ready and wear your barn clothes," she said. "Don't forget your apron."

Swiftly, I climbed up the ladder to the loft and got into my barn clothes. I grabbed an apron hanging on a nail. I felt a tug on my skirt as I ran for the door.

It was Grandma French. Her face was tense and dark. "Now Alice," she said, and there was sadness in her voice. "This is not gonna be a beautiful birth. Take this small box and blanket with you; you will need it."

I took the box and blanket, but I was not sure what Grandma was saying.

Why the box?

I had watched all the animals giving birth most of my life; I even helped Pa assist a cow birth a calf just a month ago. I knew about all the blood and all, and that birth would not be "beautiful." *For Heaven's sake*, I thought. *I know more about birthing than they realize in this house.*

Maw and I stepped up into the carriage, and away we went.

Albert drove extra fast. He instructed us, "Here you go, ladies; take these wool blankets to cover yourselves. They will keep you warm."

I brought the blanket to my face as the cool air became chill. If anyone looked at me, they saw only a blanket with two hazel eyes peering out.

The springs on the buggy bounced Maw and me all around the carriage. I held a death grip so I would not fall off.

Every time before Albert turned a sharp corner, he yelled, "*Ladies, grab onto the buggy for your life!*" As we turned, I felt gravity trying to pull us right out of the buggy towards the road.

This ride is dangerous.

Better yet, this ride is fun.

As we headed towards the shipyards of Milwaukee, we were overcome by the blackened evening fog coming up from Lake Michigan, muddled with pollution from the burning coal in the mills. It became tough to see, especially since our eyes stung.[H-1]

We stopped suddenly.

Albert helped us step down from the carriage and offered to walk us through the dark, dirty road to the alley by the brick building. We welcomed his offer; this area could be dangerous.

He walked us to the alley, where we could see the brick building. "Clara," he said to Maw. "I'll be waiting for you down the street at the end of this road. I'll be at Marty's Inn…real nice place. I can grab a meal there while I wait."

Maw said, "I will let you know if we will be here too long."

As Maw and I walked down the alley, we saw a few men sitting next to a back door on the steps of a building we were approaching. They were singing and chugging their drinks. Maw told me not to look; this just made me want to look more. Trash littered the alley. A few wild cats darted out in front of us as we walked.

The stench was awful.

In front of the building we passed, a man was caressing a lady behind a large trash barrel. Another lady was upstairs displaying her shadow out the window for the world to see. She saw the few men chugging their drinks, eyeing her. She opened the window and dangled her bare leg, swinging it back and forth. This sure got the men's attention. The woman hollered, "Do you like what you see?"

They blew back whistles.

"Then come up here, and I will show you the other leg."

I have never seen ladies act like this. I looked at Maw; she was ignoring these ladies. *What's next?*

Finally, we walked up the rusty old steps into an old brick apartment building at the end of the alley where the men were gathered. We heard a wooden door creaking on the porch as it opened.

A shadow appeared. An older woman who liked to paint her face stood at the half-opened door. She must have anticipated our arrival. I immediately started sneezing when I got close to her; she must spray herself with fragrance, so she does not have to smell the stench of where she lives.

She welcomed us in. "Clara. Good to see you, gorgeous. Come on in."

Maw started scolding her as soon as we entered. "For the grace of God, Gertie, what are you doing here? This place is filthy. Alice, watch for *rats* on the floor."

Now, this made my heart sink. I hate rodents.

Can I take this? I wondered. This was getting frightening. Would I get fearful and lose it at birth? If so, I wouldn't be much help for Maw.

Gertie quickly responded. "I don't hear you, Clara, nor do I wanna listen. Just get in here and save this poor girl. She has been laboring for days. I think her baby is coming early. Her name is Nellie."

Maw and I walked down the hall of the old house. As we went, I heard a song I recognized playing on the piano. It was a waltz called *Roses from the South*. *Well*, I thought, *at least they listen to good music here*.

Several more men and women were caressing and singing their hearts out in the main room where the piano was playing. The women had bright shiny dresses and adorned their hair with feathers. They appeared to be trying their best to lure the men into a commitment…at least for the night. The women stared at us, and the men made crude remarks as we walked on by. Maw made glaring eye contact with anyone who challenged us.

We followed Gertie through a hidden door behind a bookcase, which led us into a secret room that seemed to be a large kitchen. In the back of the kitchen was the pantry, and behind the pantry was another door that led us to a stairway.

We climbed the rickety staircase to the top floor and walked down the dark hall with uneven wooden floor planks that squeaked and made us lean as we made our way to the back room.

As we approached the end of the hall, I began to hear moans of pain. These moans penetrated my heart.

My thoughts were racing.

Will I have the strength I need? Please don't faint! What

if I throw up? How cruel. I need to keep calm. I need to be helpful. Don't faint. Be strong. Breathe deep.

Maw took a deep breath as she opened the door.

In the back of the room was a flickering light coming from an oil lamp. A foul odor tainted the air. On a beaten old bed lay a young girl not much older than Beulah, covered with blankets.

She had scraggly red hair that twisted and knotted as she thrashed herself back and forth in bed. She moaned in pain as she held her belly and couldn't seem to catch her breath.

This was Nellie.

We walked into the room and approached Nellie lying in bed. Maw said, "Nellie, we are here to help you. You can moan or cry; just don't move. I need to inspect you. We will look between your legs and see what is happening."

I was not sure if Nellie heard Maw. Her eyes were a-rolling, and her body was hot with fever.

Gertie asked Maw, "What can we do about this

fever?"

Maw told Gertie, "During the *rebellion between the states* I saw doctors use leeches to combat the bad blood; some even would drain the blood from those hot with fever. Mary, my own ma, says *bloodletting* is a temporary solution, as the red face becomes pale, and the fever may go down temporarily. But when the fever comes back, it comes back with a vengeance, as the patient is now weakened."

Gertie looked at Maw with a bit of hope. "Any leeches?"

Maw replied, "None that I know about. We must resort to cooling her down with cold washcloths and removing those heavy blankets."

Maw removed the large dirty blankets and placed a light clean blanket over Nellie, covering her for privacy. Gertie and I removed Nellie's skirt and undergarments. I kept myself from stumbling back as I took them — they smelled like rotting eggs.

Dark blood and yellow-green drainage were coming from Nellie's bottom. I gasped at the sight and regretted taking in the air.

Maw and Gertie seemed immune to this unsightly scene. They barely took in their breaths. *Could it be that not breathing deeply helps them avoid the stench?* I immediately started to breathe shallowly.

Gertie and I then brought some clean cloths dipped in cold water to place on Nellie's forehead and under her arms.

Maw asked me, "Grab the oil lamp and bring it close to the bed, as I will inspect her private place real close." I brought the lamp close, careful not to spill any oil. Maw reached into her bag and pulled out an old rag. She carefully made sure only to touch Nellie with the rag wrapped around her hand.

Through the flickering light, I could see what Maw was looking at. I saw many cuts on Nellie's birth opening, which were draining yellow-green discharge mixed with blood.

Not a good sight.

Maw must have seen my reaction and confusion. "These cuts indicate she is not having an early birth on her own," Maw said. "They're also the reason for her fever. Stay here with Nellie and hold her hand."

She threw the dirty rag in a pail next to the bed and left the room with Gertie to discuss what was happening away from Nellie.

Which left me alone with Nellie.

I could feel Nellie increasing her grip as her pains increased. I held her hand back. I was beginning to understand what Grandma French meant when she said that this birth was not gonna be beautiful.

Moments later, Maw returned with Gertie. An older lady stomped into the room with them. Maw seemed to know her. "Hulda," Maw said. "I take it this is a result of your doting care."

Hulda grunted. She seemed to have a black halo looming over her head, similar to the white halos you see in church pictures of Jesus. There was an evil presence in the room. She gave Maw and me a nasty look as she squinted her eyes and raised her upper lip.

Maw took Gertie aside to the back of the room. We could all still hear them talk.

"For Heaven's sake, Gertie," Maw said. "This girl is

not having an early baby. Someone tried to remove that baby by cutting her up to try to expel the baby. The medical profession calls this a criminal abortion."

Hulda loudly grumbled.

Maw proclaimed louder, "And a mighty sloppy one, if I say so myself."

Hulda clomped out to the hallway in a huff.

Maw joined me back at the bed and told me to grab the small blanket that we had brought from home, as the baby would be coming out soon.

We waited, and we waited…until Nellie started to make small, broken groans as a lifeless baby descended and expelled from her birth opening, covered with seething drainage.

The baby was small. Maybe the size of a three-pound sack of flour. The skin was white, covered with yellow drainage. I could see that the poor baby's skin was peeling off on its back. Parts of the lips were blackened. I couldn't tell if it was a baby boy or a girl.

I was startled at the sight of the poor thing. I tried not to look too hard. Nausea overcame me, and I started to retch. Maw gave me her stern gaze. I told myself: *Knock it off, Alice — remain still.*

Maw gently laid the lifeless baby between Nellie's legs. She pulled a roll of string from her bag, immediately tied the rope off in two places on the rope, and then cut in between the ties. Maw unapologetically ordered me, "Alice? Pick up the baby."

I exclaimed, "But Maw!" I shuddered at the thought of touching the dead baby.

Maw staunchly repeated, "Alice Ada Wood — pick up the baby now!"

My eyes filled up with tears. My heart started pounding and began to beat fast...real fast. I found it hard to breathe.

Seeing my face, Maw's expression softened just a hair. "The baby is dead, Alice. We will bring the baby home with us."

In through the nose and out through the mouth. I could

hear my grandma's words — *in through the nose and out through the mou*th.

I slowly regained composure as I deeply breathed at my grandmother's words.

I picked up the baby with rags and gently wrapped the blanket around it to cover the whole body completely. Not even the face was showing; it didn't need to.

I had held many babies before because my Maw let me go with her to visit women after the births and help with breastfeeding.

This was different. There was no life in this baby. Floppy and cool to the touch, it was a glove without a hand. I finished wrapping the poor baby and lay it gently in the box Grandma had given me. Thank goodness for Grandma French!

I stepped towards the door, holding the box. "Ok, Maw, let's go."

"Get back here; we need to wait," announced Maw.

Wait for what? I thought. Maybe that flat rope from

Nellie's bottom needed to finish coming out.

One hour later, Nellie expelled what looked like a pale, not-so-shiny red liver.

Maw massaged Nellie's tender belly soon after. Nellie did not fight, and she didn't retract from the massaging; her body was beginning to weaken. Even her moans were deteriorating.

The bleeding seemed to slow down — but then picked up in earnest. Maw pulled out a medicine bottle for the bleeding and some opium for the pain. She used a dropper to medicate Nellie. Afterward, she massaged Nellie's sore belly a bit more as Nellie softly moaned. Maw gave the medicines to Gertie.

Next, Maw pulled out a bottle labeled *Carbolic Acid* with big XXs on it from her bag and used it to wash her hands with warm water in a porcelain bowl that Gertie had brought in. She handed me the acid and told me to wash too. I hesitated. Maw reminded me, "During the war of the great rebellion, we would pour carbolic acid in the wounds to clean them and reduce the stench."

I nodded. As I washed, my hands got red and began to burn. She always said she only used carbolic acid in the worst cases.

This must have been the worst case.

After we finished washing, Maw gave me the hand balm Grandma made to soften our skin.

We walked out to the hall. Several ladies were gathered there to get an update on Nellie. Nurse Hulda sat in a corner on a big soft chair, chewing tobacco and spitting in a brass spittoon.

My Maw started trembling at the sight of her; she was seething with anger.

She started pacing back and forth.

"I am ashamed of you ladies," she said sternly. "Every one of you in the house is responsible for this young mama being so ill with fever and the death of her baby."

Nurse Hulda started to smirk. She looked beastly. She had thick chin hair and warts all over her face. As she smirked, we could see that a few of her teeth were missing. She was chugging her whiskey and chewing her tobacco like an old cow with cud between her grunts. Hulda spoke to my Maw: "That baby is a devil baby, and that is why this young mama is so sick with fever."

Maw's face and body reddened — it seemed like her rage was flowing through her veins like lava flows down a volcano. It nearly consumed her.

When my Maw talks, ladies listen, the ladies of the house listened now.

She scornfully told the ladies of the house, "We are taking this baby with us, and we will give this baby a decent burial. When Nellie dies —"

She then gazed at the women with their mouths hanging open in disbelief.

"Yes, she will die," Maw asserted.

Maw continued her rant. "When Nellie dies, I suggest you pull your money together and call the undertaker to bring Nellie up to the cemetery so that we can bury her next to her baby. God is merciful, and he will forgive her for listening to your poor

advice. As for you ladies, God be with you."
Maw glared at Nurse Hulda as she told me, "Alice, see that woman?"

"Yes, Maw."

"She is not a nurse. Just because a woman calls herself a nurse doesn't make her a nurse."

Nurse Hulda yelled at my Maw. "You got to hell, Clara!" She spat on the floor.

Oh, how I just wanted us to get out of there as soon as possible. I had never seen Maw so angry. I prayed they wouldn't start fighting like cats in a barn right in front of me.

Maw looked at Gertie. "I will not come back here, Gertie. I refuse to help those who cause their own misery. This is on you, Gertie! Clean this place up, or I'll report you."

Gertie was remorseful. "Clara, please, I don't want to lose your services. Hulda told me she was a nurse, but I now realize she cannot be trusted. Have mercy on us. I beg of you."

Maw's face softened. "Gertie, have the men wear condoms — you have more to worry about than just pregnancy. There is a sheep herder outside of town that makes them from sheep guts. I am sure he could sell you a few." Gertie nodded.

Maw continued. "And if your girls get pregnant, let them have their babies, and our church will try to find homes for them. I will send ladies from church to help you clean up your house for now."

Gertie shook her head in disbelief. "Most men won't pay for a pregnant girl."

"Not true," Maw said. "You know, Madam Stella has a place like yours on the other side of the shipyard. She says that she lets a few of her girls work when they are pregnant — making sure to hide their growing bellies. Assigning them to the most drunken customers. Often the men just pass out when their head hits the pillows."

Gertie said, "Worth giving it a try."

After another walk back down the long alley, we were delighted that Albert was waiting for us at Marty's on the main road. We gladly caught a ride with him.

Once in the carriage, I placed the box on my lap. I realized there was no life under those blankets.

In my heart, I said a quiet prayer to ask God to give me the strength to care for this deceased baby, as He was no doubt caring for its spirit in Heaven.

On the ride home, Maw explained the birth details after I asked about the rope and the liver.

"Alice, that is not a rope; it is a cord, and on the end of the cord is a placenta, not a liver. All of this feeds the baby during pregnancy. That cord was flat and wasn't as blue as I like to see. Don't let a blue baby scare you, by the way. Blue is quite normal at first. What you saw was a white baby. Without a doubt, there was no blood circulating in that baby. That baby had died long before we got there. The placenta was smaller than normal and not as shiny; it was a dusky red. Not healthy. If the baby stays in the Mama too long, the placenta can dry out and come out in chunks. I reckon her disease just started a few weeks ago as the baby was developed."

"I didn't like Hulda," I admitted.

Maw sighed. "Alice, there is often a sad and complicated story that lies behind evil people. There was a time Hulda was a decent woman and mother. Ten years ago, her husband and all five of their children were killed in a buggy accident. On the spot. So tragic...she tried midwifing for a while, but she had horrible outcomes where many of the mamas and babies died. Sadly, they died due to her lack of focus and poor practice. And, of course, a bit too much alcohol. Soon no one trusted her. Shortly after, she became known for her back-alley criminal abortions. Yet, as you can see, her problem with alcohol is impeding her judgment. She continues to practice poorly."

Finally, we got home and walked up the path to our house. Maw stopped right before the door.

"Alice, assisting with birth is hard. And this was a rough birth, and you are so young. Don't be tough on yourself."

I nodded my head in agreement. "I did not feel like I was much help today."

Maw didn't respond.

We opened the door. There stood Pa waiting for us. Without saying anything, I gave Pa the box with the unsightly baby. He was silent. He just nodded as he took the baby, walked outside, and mounted his horse. He knew what to do. *He must be used to Maw bringing home babies that have died.*

I must have looked troubled because Maw said, "Alice, don't fret. There is a place in the back of the cemetery for people to be buried that do not have money or family."

A few days later, we heard that Nellie, the baby's mama, did die. The ladies did not pay for her burial. I heard my parents say that her body was taken out to the forest. *Hopefully, she was buried,* I thought. *But maybe she was just thrown into the woods.*

When I heard this, I realized there are people who have no regard for life. I was in despair.

Several days later, as I was resting in the loft, I overheard my grandma, Beu, and my Maw conversing in the front room. Maw said, "After watching Alice at Gerties, I am not sure if she can handle childbirth. It might not be for her."

Beulah nodded in agreement. "She really is too young, Ma."

I was tired of hearing that I was too young. I decided not to say anything because I wanted to hear more.

Grandma stated, "Ladies, this wasn't a typical birth to see if Alice was good for the profession. Clara, you at least make sure Alice goes with you to attend a good birth. She deserves that."

A bit later, I walked on by Grandma, and she gave me a wink. I guess she knew I was listening.

I wanted to talk with Grandma — but not just then. I would wait until it was just Grandma and me.

A few days later, I got a good opportunity to converse with my Grandma French. We were peeling potatoes for the stew that night.

I proclaimed, "Grandma, you were right. That birth I went to was not beautiful."

Grandma nodded her head but didn't say anything.

"I was really scared having to pick up and care for that little baby that died."

Grandma finally replied. "I bet."

Grandma is always willing to listen to what I have to say. The hard part is getting her to talk.

I then asked, "Grandma, I have a question. What is an abortion?"

Grandma replied, "Did you hear women use that word at the birth?"

"Yes, I did, and I heard Maw say it too."

Grandma appeared to be sorrowful as she placed her hands on her temples. Finally, she spoke.

"Alice, most of the time, when a lady is pregnant, the little baby has time to grow until the time of birth. With an early birth, a baby can come untimely, and no one can stop it. What you are talking about is criminal abortion. Abortion is a term used by medical experts. At times, the lady does not want the baby or the pregnancy, and she may have someone try to remove the baby early. This results in the death of the baby. But, as you saw, in some cases, the mama dies too."

"Oh, Grandma," I said, "I thought it was something like that. That is so awful and very sad. You mean those mean people at Gertie's place killed that mother and her baby? I think that evil lady Hulda who said she was a nurse, did it."

"There is a lot of evil out there, Alice. Particularly with childbirth. But always remember — like I have said before, most births are beautiful, a true miracle. A gift from God. Very soon, you will bleed every month as your body gets ready to have babies too."

I knew this from Beulah, but I did not tell Grandma. Beu told me to be careful not to say anything about bleeding to our family — or in school because many homes did not talk about this. I knew this to be true, but one day I would have to say something to my friend at school Annabelle. She needed that information. *When it came to me, though,* I thought *maybe Grandma and Maw wanted to talk about this to me by themselves.*

"Are there many births this upsetting?" I asked, almost pleading. "It doesn't seem right. So much horror. I was expecting birth to be much better."

Grandma sighed. "Alice, you need to go see a beautiful birth. Has your Maw talked to you about this?"

"No. I think she may be right, though." I felt a catch in my throat. "I am not sure assisting with births is for me. It's hard. Not sure I have what it takes to help women birth. I felt I didn't do much. In fact, none of us did much; it was like we were too late."

"You know Alice, Mrs. Anderson is having her sixth baby, and her own mama recently died. So, her husband asked Maw to come. Let me talk to Maw about you going along too."

I was happy to hear Grandma would talk with Maw about this.

As I started to leave for the barn to feed the critters, I realized that I had one more pressing question to ask her. "Grandma, am I too young to attend birth?"

"It won't be your age that will hold you back from birthing."

"Okay, then — what will it be?"

"With time, you will know," answered Grandma.

I left wondering what to think. Beu says I am too young to attend a birth. Maw says I am too young to attend a birth. But Grandma says my age isn't the problem — something else is.

Why doesn't she just tell me? This was so frustrating.

I went to bed that night up in the loft and spent the evening thinking about who I was, and what I had seen during the past few days.

I didn't find any answers.

My life had changed. And soon, I would be changing too — bleeding every month, for starters. Opening the door for me to become like Maw or Grandma.

Or Nellie too.

I will not be scared, I decided. All the women I knew do this.

I prayed to God to grant me the strength to endure

this perilous life and to be strong.

Alice Ada Wood: Midwife Apprentice

CHAPTER 2
REFLECTING ON BIRTHING:
PROCESSING THE HORROR — RETURNING TO NORMALCY 1880.

Several weeks later, I was still processing Nellie's birth — and death.

How did our family get to this point in life? Are the women in our house destined to care for these feral women during birth in the untamed, lawless Midwest? Does this include me joining the women in my family by becoming a midwife?

Nellie's birth struck me. Not just the birth but the thought of living and dying in such filth.

I now realized that I had no idea of what childbirth was like, nor what kind of setting Maw and Beu usually worked in — or even what drove them to attend births day after day. I could think of easier jobs to do. It must be like Grandma said — most births are beautiful.

If this was the case, maybe — just maybe — I could give it a try.

Before I got the chance to test myself again, school had started.

Fall was ending, and I was getting ready to go back to school before the Christmas break.

One day, I just lay in my bed daydreaming.

I realized that I was so much different than I was when the last school year ended. I witnessed a ghastly birth and saw people live and work in such filthy settings.

Will my classmates know what I know? I hope not.

I imagined that one day, all these boys and girls would have children.

What does that mean?

Don't go there, Alice, I told myself.

Had I seen too much?

Eddie and I walked to school together the next morning. As usual, we stopped by to pick up my friend, Annabelle. She lived on a small farm on the road to school. She was also twelve, and I considered her my best friend.

As we approached her house, I could see Annabelle's father and brother sitting on the porch. They glared at us with suspicion.

When we were in good earshot, I asked, "Is Annabelle here?"

I didn't want to get too close to them; I've never felt comfortable around them.

Her brother spat out his chewing tobacco into a spittoon next to his chair. "She is in the house. I will go get her."

He got up and went into the house.

Her dad sat glaring at Eddie and me. "Glad you came to get her," he said. "We have a real hard time getting her to school. Her mama is so sick." His words don't match the look on his face.

Pa had told us never to go inside their home. He never said why.

Annabelle soon came out and to joined us as we walked to school.

Oh, how I wished I could help Annabelle. Even though I considered her to be my best friend, I realized I really don't know her — but what I do know is that she is troubled. Her family seemed odd to me. She was so shy and quiet; I might never know.

Later that week, it was my day to present in class. I was asked to choose my own topic. I chose to first talk about myself, then share about my family. I was a bit nervous.

We started out by reciting the Pledge of Allegiance and, of course, a prayer. That morning, Miss Violet asked, "Eddie? Have you prepared to read a scripture from our classroom Bible?"

As Eddie walked up to the front of the classroom, I noticed his head was down. He was a bit timid.

He brought the classroom Bible to the podium. As he opened it, he nervously swallowed. He probably didn't want to stutter, like he does when he is scared.

"This passage is from Isaiah 5:20: *Woe to those who call evil good and good evil, who put darkness for light and light for darkness, who put bitter for sweet and sweet for bitter.*"

He quietly sat down.

"Well done, Eddie," Miss Violet said. "I can see you were well prepared!"

Eddie smiled.

"Now, Alice, let's hear from you," announced Miss Violet.

I walked to the front of the class. I did not bring any notes; I wasn't supposed to, as requested by my teacher.

"Hello," I said. "I am Alice Wood. As you know, I am Eddie's older sister. I am medium height and have light skin. My eyes are hazel. You know, brown-green. My hair is dark brown and tends to get curly, especially when the rain and heat are in the air — just like my Pa's hair. I usually braid my hair to keep it from growing wild. Soon I will wear a corset, as Beulah, my older sister, does. Not sure what I think about that." The children in class started to giggle.

Miss Violet gave them her stern look.

I proceeded.

"My favorite outfit is my dark navy walking skirt with my cream-covered blouse with a fancy collar. I would love to have swanky black leather boots that lace up to make my outfit complete! My family and I moved here in 1880 to be near the fast-growing city of Milwaukee. My father could earn a better living here, as he is a stonecutter. While people are traveling West, we see so many women without their families. Many of them are ready to give birth. Maw and my big sister Beu answer this call to help ladies give birth in their own homes. They too, are contributing to our household funds for the family.

Frequently, we hear knocks throughout the night. Especially in the early morning. But it's a price they pay. Beu has been helping Maw with birthing since she was twelve. She is now sixteen." I glanced over to see Miss Violet's reactions; she motioned for me to continue.

"Back in Madison, we lived in a log home. My fathers' parents are from New York and moved to Madison in the 1840s. They came on a covered wagon. During the war between the states, my father was called to be a soldier in New York. This is where my parents met; they, too, came back to Wisconsin on a covered wagon. One day we hope to move out West to Tacoma or Seattle, Washington. Pa says next time; we'll take a train. No more covered wagons for our family."

I continued. "Wisconsin is known as America's Dairyland. Today we live on a very small farm close to Milwaukee, outside of the city limits. This way we can have a garden, chickens, milking cows and horses. Pa says the population explosion in Milwaukee is clogging the sewers and cesspools. It is unhealthy to live too close to those sewers. So, for now, we live close enough to the city so that Papa can easily get to work, yet far enough away to live in the country."

Miss Violet said, "Well done, Alice. Can you show the students on the classroom map where Tacoma and Seattle, Washington, are located?" She handed me her pointer stick.

"I sure can," I said and pointed them out. "As you can see, the trains mainly arrive in Tacoma as it has a better port, but my father says he believes the trains will start going North to Seattle." It was a great day, as the students did seem interested. To my surprise, a few of the students shared that their families wanted to move West too.

After school, as we walked home, Annabelle started to weep.

I told Eddie to go on ahead. He did.

"Alice," Annabelle said. "I think I am dying."

I stopped. "What makes you say that?"

She whispered. "I am bleeding — you know, down there."

I started walking again. "Oh, Annabelle, all of us girls will bleed. Hasn't your mama told you about this?"

She shook her head no.

"You are becoming a woman," I said. "Because of this, one day, you can have a baby."

I thought this would calm her. It didn't. She got more upset. As we walked up to her home, I said goodbye, and she ran up to her house in tears.

Oh, how bad I felt.

Annabelle did not go to school the next couple of days. The following week, we picked up Annabelle — and her arm was broken. My gut said someone in her family did this. Oh, how I wished I could help her. What had they done to her?

They would say her mama was sick, but we never saw her.

Where was her mama?

Alice Ada Wood: Midwife Apprentice

CHAPTER 3
STARTING A NEW YEAR:
NORMAL PHYSIOLOGICAL BIRTHING 1881

A new year had arrived.

This winter was especially brutal with all the snow we had to endure. It was like living in a never-ending blizzard.

As I lay in bed, many distractions clogged my mind. I couldn't help but think about all the work I had to do. The sound of the wind howling outside didn't help either. It reminded me of the violent winter we were experiencing. I tried my best to clear my mind and focus on getting a good night's sleep, but it was easier said than done.

Where is my school friend Anabelle? Lately, every time we stopped by her house, they told us, "*She ain't home.*"

Then there was birthing. Would I go again? I was still not sure about attending these births.

Well, that was how I felt at the moment. I would find myself changing my mind daily. I hadn't ruled it out completely.

Several weeks later, one early morning, I heard a loud knocking at our front door downstairs. Beu answered the door.

A man tenderly announced, "It is time."

It was Mr. Anderson. I recognized his voice. After he delivered the news, I heard him walk back to wait at his buggy.

Quickly, I jumped out of bed and grabbed my work clothes and an apron. I then climbed down the ladder to meet up with Maw. To my surprise, Maw was there with Beu, ready to leave without me. Had Maw forgotten about me? I was sure Grandma was going to talk with her about me coming to the next birth.

She looked surprised. "Oh, Alice. I thought I'd let you sleep, as you need to go to school."

I quickly responded, "I am ready to go!"

"Are you?"

I became hesitant…what was I saying? Just a couple of weeks ago, I was ready to give up.

But the decision was made.

I could do it. I was a Wood. We are from hardy stock. We can do hard things. I would go if Maw would let me.

Beulah said, "Take Alice, Maw. I can stay home."

Did I hear Beulah suggesting I go? Had Beulah changed? I couldn't believe my ears. I looked to Maw.

Maw called out, "All right then. Alice, grab your coat, mittens, and boots! Here is an extra scarf."

I could hardly hide my grin.

Swiftly, we ran outside with Maw's bag, met Mr. Anderson, and jumped into the buggy he had brought with him.

We were off! I was more excited than scared this time. I knew the Andersons, and they were a kind family.

What would a normal birth look like? What would I do to help Maw? It would be so exciting to see a little baby born.

How fun…or wait a minute, could it be a bad experience?

I would not go there, I decided. I need to keep up with good thoughts.

We took the buggy through the snow. It was the wee hours of the morning. A rising sun began to light the trail. As we approached the Anderson home, I could see a burning candle in a window. Smoke was rising from the chimney.

Once we arrived, I followed Maw and Mr. Anderson as we ran up and entered the home. The glowing embers softly lit the living room. I gazed at the back of the room towards the kitchen. The darkness impaired my vision, but I could hear the faint sounds of a woman breathing.

As I got nearer, I could see it was Mrs. Anderson, rocking her hips as she leaned on the kitchen table. Between contractions, she was kneading dough. Focusing on getting that bread ready for her family before the baby comes, I imagined. As she began to knead harder, she started to breathe deeper, blowing in and out through her mouth.

I thought that she better stop this and get ready to birth. *Should I step in?*

I wanted to be helpful, so I stepped forward and said, "Mrs. Anderson, I can…"

But I wasn't sure what I could do.

Maw pulled me back and gave me a nod. "Alice. Mrs. Anderson is doing just fine."

Why doesn't Maw want me to help Mrs. Anderson? I was so baffled.

All the Anderson children were nearby, on the enclosed back porch. They were playing board games on the floor.

So early to be playing games, I thought. Perhaps this distracts them from hearing their mother's gentle moans of pain.

The eldest Anderson child, Seth, greeted his father. After a brief exchange, Seth grabbed the three younger boys and headed out the door to spend the day at the neighbor's home.

Charlene, their oldest daughter, remained in the house. She was close to my age. This would be the second birth of a sibling she would attend.

Maw had told me that none of the Anderson children went to a formal school. They did all of their schooling at home.

Mr. Anderson showed Maw what they already had prepared. "Clara, here is a packet of fresh-off-the-press newspapers. I made sure to bake these cheesecloths in the oven. Over there is a bottle of carbolic acid."

Mr. Anderson seemed ready. He had a large pot of water boiling on the stove. He poured the hot boiling water into his copper bed warmer. Then he walked into the bedroom and placed it under the blankets in their bed to warm up. He alternated the copper bed warmer with warm embers from the fireplace placed in a metal pan on the end of a pole. He would repeat this task several times throughout the night. This way, his wife could lie in a warm cozy bed after the baby came. He was so thoughtful and devoted.

Maw called me and Charlene over. "I will show you how to prepare the living room for the birth," she said. "First, we drape the newspapers over there on this couch. As you can see, Mr. Anderson melted wax on them to protect the couch. The wax allows the blood to roll off. The heat from the press makes newspapers clean. Then, be sure to cover the couch with those cheesecloths. With the cheesecloth, we can collect debris, which is then easy to remove and throw away. Use that bucket over there. In my bag, we have a bunch of clean rags. Those can go to this wash bucket if we feel we can wash them. Otherwise, place them in this trash bucket. After the floor is clean, in this house, we can use the carbolic acid to sprinkle on the floor to reduce the stench."

We then all went to the sink to wash our hands with soap.

"Now girls, not just your hands, wash up to your elbows," Maw reminded us.

The house was big, but there was just one room in the main area of the house. Behind that room was Mr. and Mrs. Anderson's bedroom. The main room consisted of a kitchen on one side and a gathering room on the other side with a big table in the middle. Clean as could be.

Maw explained to us that the birth would happen in the gathering room, on or near the couch. Then after, as the bleeding slowed down, Mrs. Anderson would transfer to her back bedroom.

Mr. Anderson opened a cabinet under the sink. "This is where the oil is to refill the lanterns, and right outside the back door is extra wood for the stove."

Mr. Anderson was so helpful; he never left his wife's side.

Maw pulled a dozen sanitary pads Grandma French had made from her bag. They all had cheesecloth over them, fastened with one stitch on top of each one to keep off any debris. She handed Charlene and me two little knives. "You may need these to break open packets or to remove the cheesecloth from the pads."

Then, Maw walked over to the rocking chair and started knitting.

Guess we were waiting. I noticed that Charlene seemed more at home in the situation than I was.

Later, I walked outside with Maw to pick up more wood.

Maw told me the important thing was to be there for Mrs. Anderson while still allowing the birth to transpire on its own time. "See how Mrs. Anderson relaxes, and if she gets uncomfortable, she will seamlessly change her position; this facilitates the baby to be able to move down the birth canal."

This went along with Maw and Grandma's mantra: *Move the Mom, Move the Baby.*[B-1]

Mr. Anderson carried over what looked like a fancy chamber pot — a wooden stool with a hole in it, emptying into a bucket. He had made it himself out of wood. He was so clever. Mrs. Anderson sat on this for nearly an hour. I was wondering if she was having trouble defecating. Yet, she seemed comfortable, and continued to rock right on the stool.

Slowly, Mrs. Anderson walked over to her spinning wheel. She sat on her 3-legged chair. Again, during contractions, I could see her rocking in a rotating manner, and taking in big breaths, then slowly blowing out.

Watching Mrs. Anderson's birth was a beautiful sight. I was in awe.

I watched her respond to her baby inside her belly as they both worked together to accomplish this miraculous feat called birth. If she felt uncomfortable, she changed her position.

At the right time, Mr. Anderson carefully assisted his wife over to the couch, where she knelt on the seat leaning towards the back. She kept rocking, lifting one knee at a time. She sighed and exhaled as the contractions increased. I could hear soft moans.

Soon, she became quiet and laid down on the couch to take a rest.

What was happening?

I would react to this unexpected action, but as I watched Maw continue to knit and Mr. Anderson just walked over to reload the stove with wood and boil more water, I realized all was well.

One hour later, Mrs. Anderson was energized after her rest. She repositioned herself back to kneeling on the couch and started to push. She announced, *"It's coming."*

After softly blowing air in and out, she gave out a loud moan as she started pushing out her baby.

Maw quietly positioned herself to catch the baby. Immediately, as the baby was birthed, a gush of fluid bathed the baby, and Maw too. Maw reached behind Mrs. Anderson's legs and lifted up the baby. Mrs. Anderson rolled onto her back, and Maw helped her position the baby on her chest.

The baby gurgled a bit. Initially, he looked a bit blue, but I saw him quickly pink up as Maw vigorously dried him off. He let out a blustering cry.

Pure joy filled the room.

"It's a boy!" confirmed Maw.

"He is so awake!" I declared as I saw him gaze around the room. Maw placed a dry warm blanket on him to keep him covered on the warm chest of his mother.

Maw gazed at the cord. What was she looking for, I thought. I grabbed the roll of string and scissors as I walked over to help. Maw gently leaned over to me and said, "Not yet."

So, we waited more.

I watched Maw grab the cord, and she nodded her head as the cord became lighter in color. She then grabbed the string this time and made two very tight ties on the cord near the baby's belly. Then, she cut between the strings. The knotted cord continued to hang out of her birth opening.

We wait. Again.

I noticed the cord getting longer.

I saw a gush of blood. I was worried.

We waited.

Then, certain enough, the liver — placenta — was expelled.

Maw grabbed the placenta and placed it in a bowl. She then reached up and massaged Mrs. Anderson's belly. She asked, "Charlene and Alice? Come feel how hard the uterus is now; it is firm as a coconut."

So, she was not massaging the belly, as I thought. There was a hard ball in there called a uterus.

Maw took my hand, and we applied firm pressure to the top of the uterus and watched the bleeding subside. Then, Maw had me apply constant pressure for two minutes. She said, "It is the best 2-minute investment you can make. It will reduce bleeding and keep the uterus firm." [B-2]

Following that, she had me look at the placenta to see that it was intact. She noted there were no missing pieces.

We looked at the shiny side that had a broken bag attached. Maw told us this was the bag where the baby lived while it grew. We could see the lumpy and bumpy parts on the other side of the placenta. This part was attached to the mama inside the uterus, which grew with the baby. After the birth, the large uterus is what we massage; it contracts and causes the bleeding to subside.

All this happened while Mrs. Anderson was feeding her baby with her breast and smiling at him.

This was what Grandma French was talking about. Birthing was indeed beautiful.

I looked up at Mr. Anderson and saw that he had a tear in his eye. He proclaimed, "This is our fifth son; we shall call him Quentin." Mrs. Anderson and Charlene's eyes were glowing with happiness as Mr. Anderson gave him his name.

Maw pulled me aside and said, "Let's get to work finishing that bread Mrs. Anderson was making and cleaning up the area."

We got to work. Charlene joined us.

Later, I noticed that Mr. Anderson was reloading the copper tin with more boiling water to heat the bed. Next, he walked over to hold Quentin and stroke his cheeks. He handed Quentin to Charlene to hold as well.

Maw and I helped Mrs. Anderson clean up and fitted her with new pads that Grandma made with cheesecloth, along with a lovely clean gown. Then, Mr. Anderson passed Quentin for me to hold.

This was the highlight of my day.

I was amazed at how clean the baby was, with his skin so soft with such a fresh smell of a new baby. He had little white hairs on the top of his head and small white dots on the tip of his nose.[B-3]

So cute.

Mr. Anderson helped Mrs. Anderson to urinate in the wooden pot he had constructed. Then, he helped her walk down to their bedroom.

I brought Quentin to her as she snuggled under the blankets in their warm and cozy bed.

We both hugged Mrs. Anderson before we left; she was so grateful for our help. Charlene expressed her gracious thanks too.

Mr. Anderson walked with us to the gathering room and said goodbye. He handed Maw an envelope. She told him we could walk home, as it was only three miles away. And that we could return the next day to follow up and see if there was anything else we could do.

Mr. Anderson said, "Thanks, but we will be all right. I can take it from here, ladies; this is my sixth baby."

Initially, I was disappointed that Maw offered to walk. It was three miles in knee-high snow.

Not fun.

But it was beautiful.

While Quentin was being born, the Heavens had opened, and a fresh layer of glistening snow covered the landscape.

I had so many questions about the birth to ask Maw as we strolled through the sparkling snow.

I first asked her, "Why did you wait to cut the cord?"

"Did you see me feel the cord pulsating?"

"Yes, I did."

"Well then, Alice," said Maw. "As you could see, I was feeling for a beat. The beat in the cord lets me know that the placenta was pumping blood through the cord to the baby. There was a lot of blood in that placenta that the baby could use. We need to wait for the cord to finish pumping."

I was baffled. "But Maw. You did not wait with Nellie."

"True, Alice, but Nellie's baby had died."

Oh, of course.

I probed more. "Why did you not want me to help Mrs. Anderson as she prepared to bake her bread? It would have been so helpful for her."

"Making and focusing on the bread is a way Mrs. Anderson can distract herself from the pains of birthing. Also, it's a way for her to express love and care for her family before the baby arrives."
I then inquired, "I have heard you and Grandma always say, when birthing, *'Bring the baby down to the ground, then up to the sky.'*[B-4] But I did not see you do that with Mrs. Anderson. You first took the baby to the sky!"

Maw chuckled. "Oh, Alice, you are so smart. Did you see that with the birth today that she was on all fours? I reached behind the mother. We must adjust to the position of the mother. When a woman is lying on her back and not moving, the baby's head can cause pressure against the pubis, which can result in the woman tearing and hamper her ability to urinate. However, when the mom is on all fours, the baby comes out easier. Did you notice we did not use the carbolic acid to wash our hands?"

"Yes, I did. I also heard you specify in this home to only use on the floor to reduce the stench."

"Yeah, I did not want you washing your hands with it," chuckled Maw. "Like I've told you before, we used it to wash hands and pour in wounds in the war of the rebellion. But there was a lot of filth and gangrene in those dirty hospitals."

"Yeah, in Gertie's house too!"

She nodded and patted my shoulder.

What an interesting day.

I learned so much by being there and helping with the birth. There was so much to learn, and I was so eager to learn more. It was even fun. I could hardly wait to tell Grandma.

Soon, spring was in the air. Much like birth, we saw an awakening. New life had arrived: budding flowers readying to bloom, the birds singing their songs as they strived to attract a mate, the bees buzzing to pollinate the plants and flowers. Warmer days waited for us. The sun would warm the ground, and our days would be longer.

Eddie and I walked to school every morning after we did our chores. I collected the eggs, then Eddie and I shared feeding the critters. Beulah milked the cows every morning. This had to be done by 8 o'clock so we could get to school by 9 o'clock.

Miss Violet our schoolteacher, was new. She was very strict, and I didn't understand her discipline.

We had a boy in my class named Thomas who often disobeyed. Miss Violet always sat him in the corner with a big white cone hat with a 'D' on it. They call this a dunce hat. I guess she thought this would make him more obedient. It didn't.

This week, Miss Violet drew a circle on the big slate board in front of the class and made him stick his nose in it for one hour. I am not sure what he did wrong, as I don't like to stare.

My favorite subject was reading and writing. The youngest kids sat in the front row. When other students were being drilled. I would go down to the little children, who sat in the front of the class and help them write or recite their ABCs until it was time for the teacher to drill me and see if I could recite a passage from a book or the Bible. We used the Bible in class because most of our families have a Bible at home that we could use to practice reciting and reading.

Eddie and I only went to school in winter and spring, from November until May. Most kids in our school did the same. Only about half the kids ever showed up. We brought our lunch in a pail and shared a tin cup to share water. We have *nooning* for one hour, during which we eat our lunch.

The school was encouraging us to start the summer program in June until early September. I might consider doing that. I doubt Eddie would, as he liked helping Pa and going fishing in the Summer.

One day as Eddie and I walked to school, we reluctantly decided to check on Anabelle again. We hadn't seen her for months.

Oh, how we dreaded going up to that door.

We knocked on the broken door. Her father stomped up to us. This time, he was belligerent and very drunk; he slurred his words.

"What are you kids doing here? Anabelle will not be going to school anymore. More importantly, don't stop by here anymore."

As we left, I glanced back. I saw Anabelle looking through the window behind the curtain. She had a black eye.

Several months later, we saw Annabelle in town shopping. I could see she was with child. She walked away and acted like she did not know who I was.

I was distraught. Pregnant and just thirteen years old.

Who fathered her baby? What would her life be like? Soon, her family moved away. I missed having a friend my age; I would always worry about her.
I am grateful for my loving family. It was times like this, that I appreciated my parents and grandparents.

Maw had demonstrated how she cleverly cared for women and their babies, particularly during birth. She was skilled; she knew when and why to use her skills. I couldn't help but feel she knew exactly how a pregnant woman's body worked, especially during birth. She had learned from the best — her mother Grandma French, who learned from her mother, and so on and so on.

In addition, she learned a lot when she cared for wounded Union soldiers in New York and Pennsylvania during the war. I could see how she applied her knowledge, from her days working in field hospitals, of washing hands and preventing gangrene or pus-producing wounds to the women she took care of.

Even today, Maw and Grandma made a point to attend many of the hospital presentations in Milwaukee. There were no books for us to use. They listened to doctors and others who came from big places like New York City to hear their stories of healthcare and birthing. They especially prioritized speakers from New York State, where they were both from.

Beu was still my Maw's best helper. They were both so busy. I got to attend the births and assisted only when school was out. Maw was always telling me, "School first, Alice."

But Beu was hiding a secret. She told me, in confidence, that she didn't really like helping with birthing. It's not that she hated it, but it was just not her favorite thing to do. She never told Maw or Grandma about this; she didn't want to disappoint them. After all, they both love birthing, and it's a big part of their culture.

I wouldn't tell either. It was not my place.

Lately, I'd noticed that many people are moving west without their extended families. It was not a good thing, as women can feel scared when giving birth without the support of their loved ones. It was always helpful to have a few aunties, sisters, or even grandmas around to lend a helping hand. That's why I'm here for those ladies and their families, just like my Maw would be.

My father, Pierson, fought in the great rebellion alongside his two younger brothers, Benjamin and Albert. Unfortunately, Uncle Benjamin was shot in the face at just fifteen years old during the war. To hide his injury, he liked to wear a beard. Both of Pierson's brothers currently resided in Kansas.

During the war, Pa met Maw in Gettysburg, Pennsylvania. Maw and her sisters helped soldiers who were injured in the war. Pa had been shot in the leg. War doctors – *sawbones* – wanted to cut his leg off — but my Maw wouldn't let them. She not only saved his leg, but she saved his life.

Maw dressed his wounds with salve she had made from the excrement of cows. She said this secret ingredient fought diseases of the flesh and bones.[B-5]

My father always spoke highly of my mother, describing her as the most remarkable woman he had ever encountered. He often praised her intelligence and beauty. When he brought her out west to Wisconsin in a covered wagon, he knew he needed a strong and resilient partner. And my mother was exactly that — tough as nails and unbreakable.

Pa and his father before him were both stonecutters, and Pa learned the trade as an apprentice with his own father. In fact, my grandfather was once contacted by the governor of Wisconsin to carve a stone representing Wisconsin's statehood, and that stone eventually became a part of the Washington Monument in Washington D.C. It was incredible to think about the history behind such a beautiful monument.

My family gave me strength in this untamed wild west.

Susan E. Fleming

Wood Family Immigration Story

Like thousands of other American families, the Wood family took part in the *Westward Expansion*. As immigrants from Northern Europe, they fled oppression from nobles. Soon, their ancestors colonized the eastern shores of what would become the United States. Settling in cabins in western New York, the Woods found their homes being destroyed during the *French-Indian Wars*. In a short time, they found themselves fighting their fathers in a *Revolutionary War*. Shortly after, they fought their brothers in a bloody Civil War, which gave birth to an industrialized nation and ended slavery, although at a terrible cost.

The *American Civil War* went by many names during and immediately post-war: War of the Great Rebellion, War Between the States, and War Between Brothers. Frederick Douglas referred to it as the Abolition War, Slaveholder's Rebellion, and the Freedom War. Publicly, in the 1890s, it became known as the Civil War.

The Wood family was a microcosm of the nation as it expanded West. All this westward expansion happened in less than 120 years. Babies were born this entire time, of course. Also, illnesses spread, and injuries happened, leading to those deaths that occurred. Schools were created and laws were enacted. Americans, rebellious by nature, did not want to be told what to do.

But they were told.

The Woods continued to move west to the newly created Wisconsin Territory, then on westbound to Seattle, where again they tried to create a new life free from tyrants and oppression.

CHAPTER 4
BIRTHING:
ACROBATICS
MILWAUKEE - 1882

Finally, Beu had told Maw and Grandma that she didn't want to be a midwife.

I decided to take on more responsibilities when Beu started to cut back on her workload. I was eager to learn and expand my skills, so I took on the challenge even though I was only fourteen years old. It was a valuable learning experience that helped me grow and develop as a midwife.

I soon realized that sometimes pardoning ourselves for not having all the answers was okay. What was more important was that I would keep trying and persevering. I desired to learn different skills to help mothers and babies during birthing. I knew it was normal to have doubts but not to let them hold me back from moving forward and pursuing my goals.

After all, everyone who had helped with birthing must have started somewhere.

First, I had to acknowledge that I lacked experience. I realized this was not what Grandma had meant when she said it was not my age that would hold me back. Hence, being young means you lack experience. Wisdom. At this point, I was still trying to find out what was holding me back.

Maw constantly reminded me always be attentive. She always told me that when I started thinking this is just a routine birth, that's when something would go wrong. Missing a small subtle clue can lead you in the wrong direction.

What were the subtle clues that I could miss, I wondered? But when I asked, I always got the same answer:

You will know or "Could be."

I found this very unsatisfying!

Maw told me always remember there are two people sharing space in that pregnant body trying to complete this feat called childbirth. They are not only connected by a cord, but they also share nutrients, air, and blood. Even more so, their spirits are connected, and it is in the womb that the baby first feels love.

There was a lot to remember. By this point, though, I did have some things down. I opened my journal and took note:

In the early stages of labor, it was a good idea to keep the mom active and moving around. You could suggest activities like walking or rocking in a chair or stool. If a rocking chair was not available, a three-legged stool can work well too. The key was to help the mom find a comfortable position that would allow her to listen to her body and her baby. By staying connected to her body, she will be able to sense when it is time to push and give birth. Remember to encourage and support her every step of the way.

During birth, it was important to be mindful of the contractions that will expand and contract the uterus, as they facilitate the baby's descent and eventual expulsion. Applying gentle pressure to the fetal head during delivery may help prevent tears near the urethra, but not necessarily near the rectum.

Additionally, it was worth noting that providing support and comfort to the mother throughout the birthing process is crucial. It was also common to use warm washcloths on the mother's bottom unless there was swelling, in which case cool cloths may be more appropriate. As the baby rotates down and out, it was helpful to bring the baby down to the floor and then up to the sky. It was interesting to observe the baby's head during delivery, as it initially appears somewhat like knuckles on a hand, but then transforms into a perfectly round shape upon emerging. It was truly a remarkable experience.

These are just the basics.

Above all, Maw stressed, look for clues, and look for cues. What clues or cues? Will I ever get this right? I probed Maw. She told me a cue was just a hint, whereas a clue was an actual information piece. To me, their meaning seemed to be overlapped.

One afternoon, after I walked in the door from school, Grandma pulled me aside and asked if I could help.

Apparently, Maw had left to help with a birth two hours prior. But just an hour ago, a young man named Jakob Zimmerman stopped by to ask for help for his wife, Ana, who was ready to birth. They had just arrived from Germany to help with a local brewery. So, they didn't know many people in town.

I'd have to go by myself. Grandma told me it wouldn't be too tough — and anyway, Maw would be along as soon as she could.

I agreed to go.

I set out to the Zimmerman home on horseback, grateful for Grandma's help and guidance. I made sure to bring the larger bag we had put together for new mothers, as advised, and hoped that I could assist the overwhelmed couple. Knowing that Maw would be arriving soon to provide additional support was reassuring.

I ran out to the barn and mounted our horse, Sadie. She was our oldest horse, but she had a good gait, and more importantly, she listened.

Would Maw be able to help me in time? I am NOT ready to attend a birth on my own.

I approached the flats owned by the brewery for their workers. Most of the young workers lived there. They stayed there for little rent.

I dismounted Sadie and tied her to a long post. I soon found building H.

Well, here I went. What would be, would be.

I headed upstairs to the second-floor flat, 2-F. As I walked down the hall and approached the rooms, I heard the faint sound of someone in distress. It seemed like a woman in labor. It was clear that privacy was not a priority in this building.

A label on the door read Herr Zimmerman. *Good — I am at the right place.* I knocked on the door, and a young man answered.

"*Zehr gut.* You must be Clara. You are much younger than I imagined!"

I answered, "No, Clara was out. I am Alice, her daughter and apprentice." Jakob appeared a bit uncomfortable but let me in. I walked inside, and there was a woman who must have been Ana in the main room.

Jakob confirmed my guess. "This is my wife, Ana. Is there anything I can do to help?"

I reached into my bag and pulled out a copper pot. I handed it to Jakob. "Yes," I answered him. "Make sure you keep the room warm and start boiling water for this pot right away. Fill the pot often, as we will use it to warm your bed. After the birth, we can tuck Ana and the baby into a cozy warm bed."

Ana was swaying in Jakob's rocking chair recently made for her. I asked her, "How do you like the chair?"

I saw she had a big grin between her painful contractions. I assured them that the chair was a good place for Ana to be.

I brought with me the extra big birthing bag.

I prepared the couch for birthing. I dripped wax over

the newspapers, then I draped them over the couch. I then pulled out a roll of cheesecloth and laid it over the wax-dripped newspapers on the couch. I had come to like how cheesecloth was good at picking up debris. Together, the newspapers and cheesecloth would do a great job of protecting the couch.

Several hours later, Ana had a good rhythm of breathing and blowing. As the labor pains increased, she started to breathe deeper, blowing in and out through her mouth. Her moans became stronger.

A gush of liquid came out of her birthing passage. It was clear. Again, I washed my hands and forearms with soap.

I asked Ana a few times if she would like to move. But to my surprise, Ana chose to stay on the rocker for the entire birth. She just increased the rocking when the painful contractions came. We never used the couch. Jakob placed a pillow under each of her arms.

In three hours, I could see the baby's head protruding. I got down on the floor and placed gentle pressure on the baby's head.
I noticed that Ana was beginning to bleed. A little

bleeding was normal — but this seemed like more bleeding than I had seen before. Plus, the baby was having a slower descent.

I began to worry.

But worrying doesn't get the job done.

Right?

Wait, are these clues or cues?

Excessive bleeding — slow descent.

Okay — I got the cues, but what does this mean? Where was Maw? What should I do?

Ana called out with a moan, "It's coming! Whew, whew, whew. This is more than I can bear!"

"Breathe with me, Ana. In through the nose — out through the mouth…breathe for your baby; you can do it. Jacob, bring that rolling pin over here and roll it on her back."

Remember — during expulsion, baby down to the ground and up to the sky. So important. Here comes the baby, wait – wait, it was not ready to come out...

I felt tension. Another contraction came with more blood.

Oh no, I thought, *I can't bring the baby down.* The baby wasn't coming out.

Think fast, Alice.

Slowly the baby emerged but didn't come out very far. I had no choice but to place its head on Ana's right upper thigh as it flipped.

Oh my! It looked like that baby did a somersault. I had kept the baby close to Ana's thigh as I felt tension with the cord. I began to dry the baby off. Good to see the baby was slowly pinking up as I felt the cord starting to pulsate more.

Okay, here comes the placenta! I thought.

That was quick — less than 15 minutes. I placed the placenta full of blood between Ana's legs, next to the baby.

This works.

Oh yes…one more thing!

I called out. "It's a boy!

Jakob smiled a huge smile standing next to Ana. "We should name him Fritz, like your father, Ana."

I could see Ana was pleased by the loving smile on her face.

I remembered that I needed to place the baby on the mom's chest. Since the placenta was still attached, I could feel the beat. It was still pumping blood to the baby. I did not want to cut the cord.

But the cord was short.

Hmmm. I can move them together. The warm placenta will keep the baby warm.

I like this.

As I moved them together to Ana's chest, I made sure to stimulate the baby as I dried him off. He pinkened up as his breathing became less gurgled.

Finally, the baby let out a gigantic cry! Cries of joy

filled the room.

Then, I massaged her uterus. I placed gentle pressure on the uterus until I noticed it was firming up.

Ana lovingly stroked her baby. "Jakob, we did it. We have a baby."

I looked at little Fritz as he started scooting to Ana's breast to feed. I helped them attach.

Soon, the cord stopped pulsating.

Next?

Oh yeah.

I grabbed the string roll from the bag, made two ties on the cord close to the baby's belly, and then made the cut. I placed the placenta in a bowl that Jakob had brought in. I would inspect it later.

I waited as the new little family got to know each other to keep an eye on Ana's bleeding — and of course, Fritz.

After about an hour, Jakob handed me Fritz to help Ana to an older rocker in which he had cut a hole in the bottom. This allowed for the urine to empty into a bucket he had placed underneath the seat. Then, he helped Ana to their cozy warm bed.

I followed them into their bedroom and handed Jakob back their baby while I checked Ana's belly.

I instructed him. "Jakob, see how I massage her belly? We call the organ the baby grows in a uterus. That's what I'm massaging. Come feel how it gets hard, like a coconut. It might first get bigger, then it should come down by tomorrow. Gently massage it a couple of times a day until the bleeding subsides."

As the family spent time in the bedroom, I walked out to the living room and begin to clean the room.

Jakob had left me a big bucket to place any rubbish into. There was a lot.

I threw away the old rags I used for drying and the unused newspaper that I used to gather the blood and debris off the floor. Then, I threw it all in the bucket. I mopped the floor. I then went to the sink and washed my hands with soap.

Finally, I gathered my supplies and tried to quietly slip out the door. Jakob caught me; he asked me to wait and then joined me. He shook my hand as he handed me an envelope. I'd contribute most of this money to the family fund.

It was late at night when I walked outside — and there was Sadie waiting for me. She neighed. She was ready to get home. I mounted her for my ride home.

She picked up her gait as we got closer to home; she was barn sour.

I took the trail near the river as it was easier to see. I didn't see any people on the trail, but I did hear the owls.

As I rode home, I had time to contemplate Ana's birth. Overall, the mom and baby did very well.

But did I do everything right?

I was looking forward to talking with Maw and asking her a few questions.

Soon I was home. I dismounted Sadie, removed her saddle and blanket, and brushed her down. I then took off her bridle and opened the pen. I could see that hay was already waiting for her in her feeding box. Very thoughtful of Eddie or Beulah.

It was late. Real late. I walked into our house, and there was Maw. She had just arrived home from her own birth that she had attended.

We had a good laugh as we were both too busy with our own births to have any concerns about the other. Moreso, we were both exhausted. We both decided to go to bed and talk in the morning.

I slept in the next morning until after breakfast. I missed school. Beu and Eddie took care of the chores. After I woke up and dressed, I walked into the kitchen and met Maw. Grandma was there too.

We spent the next hour discussing Ana's birth.

"This mama was bleeding more than usual as the baby descended," I told them. "What could be the reason for that?"

Maw nodded. "That extra bleeding during labor was probably due to the cord, which was most likely short and was pulling the placenta off as the baby descended."[6.]

"I believe you are right, Maw!"

I told her and Grandma, "I felt helpless as the baby came down. The only thing I could do was to keep the head close to Ana's upper thigh. Then it looked like the baby did a somersault!"

Grandma and Maw both burst out laughing!

"*Looked* like a somersault?" Grandma laughed. "Most likely he *did do* a somersault in an attempt to keep the short cord intact!" They had both experienced this themselves.

Ah — the cues.

Bleeding and slow descent could be a short cord. Or? Why didn't I figure this out?

I had just begun to feel I did a good job. Let's hope I can continue to feel this way.

I asked them, "So the bleeding and slow descent meant a short cord, right."

"Could be," Maw responded.

I had heard that before, and it was always unwelcome. This 'could be' mentality really made this work so frustrating. I shook my head as I walked away.

Maw and Grandma chuckled as they saw that I was frustrated.

More time passed, and birthing was going well. In fact, I attended four more births over the next two months. I was feeling a bit more confident.

Now, I needed to place my focus on high school. Or so Maw and Grandma said.

I wanted to leave school this year because I was too busy with birthing — and I wasn't learning anything at school to help me with that.

School was so repetitive and took too much of my time. Most girls my age had stopped going to school by fifteen; some girls I knew were already married. It won't be long, and I will be fifteen.

Nevertheless, Maw and Grandma always said no, end of the story, when I proposed leaving school. They had their own ideas of me attending a nursing school. Beulah got to leave school at fifteen, but not me.

The only saving grace at school, was that I did love to write.

Months later, a family with a girl named Johanna moved into our school. I was especially excited about this since she was my age. Her family had recently immigrated from Germany. Her dad was the new Brewmeister of the brewery closest to our home. Like our family, they chose to live outside the city to have a place to raise animals and kids.

At first, we spent every day at nooning eating lunch, and talking as much as we could, given her limited English.

Slowly, she began to learn English. I didn't mind that we couldn't talk about everything yet. It was just nice to have someone other than my little brother Eddie to sit with me. Eddie was happy, too, since her two younger brothers were great fun for him during lunch. They shared their kaleidoscopes to peek through with him and their favorite games of hide and seek and walking on stilts. Johanna and I would occasionally join them, as it looked like so much fun.

We were lucky that our school had so many activities for all of us during nooning. This was a win-win for Miss Violet, as we would be tired and ready to sit and do our schoolwork.

Soon, Johanna and I were able to understand each other. One afternoon at lunch, Johanna inquired,

"Alice, vat do you want to do when you get older? Do you vant children?"

I replied, "I hope one day to have a family and children, but not right away. I might even go to a college one day. Right now, I assist my Maw with helping women birth in their homes."

"Alice dat is wunderbar; you must be very brave." Johanna then shared, "I am learning how to sew mit meine mutter."

I responded, "Nice; I would love to see what you have done."

Johanna lit up. "One day, I will have you come to my haus."

We both agreed that would be lots of fun.

At last, I loved going to school again. Friends made such a difference. I decided I would look at school as a time to develop my writing skills.

Johanna invited me to her home several times, but helping with births always was in my way.

I started wishing Maw didn't depend on me so much.

CHAPTER 5
REFINING THE CRAFT:
"NOT THE HEAD — THEN WHAT?"
MILWAUKEE - 1884

It had taken many years of birthing before my confidence grew.

Yet, Maw constantly reminded me that every birth was unique and that even she was continuously learning and expanding her knowledge of birth.

At the same time, I was maturing myself and becoming a woman. I was sixteen years old. A couple of years ago, I had my first bleed. Today, I could say I am a woman capable of making a baby.
I often dreamed about having a baby that I could call my own. However, I did not desire or feel ready to be married.

At times I was a young woman who embraced what it meant to be a woman, who was very different from a man physically and emotionally. I came to believe women were particularly strong and highly tolerant of pain as I watched them endure birth. Women also have many innate qualities that add to this, such as empathy, gentleness, and kindness as they tend to their new babies.

Yet, I sometimes feared what being a woman meant to others. Would I attract men who were good to me like my father was to my mother or even like Mr. Anderson was to his wife? Complimenting each other and setting common goals to achieve during our lives? Or would I attract a man who looked at me as an object to fulfill his desires?

Did I have the skill to know the differences?

All I knew was I didn't right then. I wasn't ready.

Finally, I had time to go to Johanna's house. We decided to walk home together after school.

At the river bend, Eddie took a turn and headed home. Johanna, her little brothers, and I started up a hill. We walked up to an impressive ranch home.

Johanna asked me to wait on the porch while she went inside. The porch had a wooden rocker on it. I sat down, started to rock, and took in the beautiful view of the rolling hills.

In the distance, I could see a young man walking up from the barn. He had an interesting face; he was good-looking, even if he was unshaven. He was tall and handsome. As he got closer, I could see his green eyes sparkled. I was careful not to stare. I wondered if he worked here on the farm.

"Hallo — are you here visiting?" he said, with a German accent.

"Yes, I am. I am here with Johanna. She is inside." I replied.

"Zehr gut," he said. He then walked over to the corral to feed the horses.

Johanna came out to get me. "Come inside and meet my mother. She doesn't speak much English." As we entered the house, there she was, standing in the main room near her kitchen. Johanna introduced us, "This is my mother, Mrs. Lanfer. Mama, das ist meine Schulfrendin Alice."

She greeted me with open arms and a big smile.

Her mother was so gracious; she gave me a grand tour of her home. Her favorite place was the kitchen. She had a large oven fed with coal and a large table to prepare her food. She had an ice box to preserve her food by keeping it cold. She even had running water with a sink.

We then walked into the gathering room. Her mother showed me her prized possession from Germany: a wooden German clock with a little bird that came out of two little wooden doors at the hour and cuckoos. Just like a live little bird! She shared, "Mein Vater gab mir das, als wir mit einem Schiff von Deutschland nach Amerika fuhren."

I nodded my head, as I knew enough German to understand. Mrs. Lanfer said, *my father gave this to me when we took a ship from Germany to America.*

I followed Johanna to her room, where she opened the top of a sturdy wooden chest. She called it her *hope chest*. One day she hoped to have a family. She displayed her detailed sewing pieces. "Alice come here; I vant you to see vat I have sewed."

"Lovely; you have worked hard to make these. Aww, is this a baby bib and outfit?"

"Yes, it is. I like knitting too. Look at these booties I am making."

"I love knitting too; I would love to see how you knit these booties."

We heard her mother call us. We went back to the kitchen to assist her. She had spent the day getting a tasty stew ready for the evening supper at the end of the day. Like most families on the farms, they had a larger afternoon dinner right after noon. I went out to help Johanna set the dining table. We set the table with eight places. I asked if anyone else was coming to supper, and she said no, just her family and me. After we finished helping her mother prepare plates, we walked them out to the dining room.

Everyone was soon seated.
Including the young man, I had met outside.

Johanna then introduced me to her family. "This is my father, Herr Lanfer, and my two older brothers, Alfred and Josef, and of course, you know my little brothers."

Ah, so the handsome young man was her brother, Josef.

I made sure to sit closer to Johanna and her mother, as I didn't want to come off too flirtatious.

The dinner discussion was lively. They discussed their day and brought in their views of the presidential candidates, James Blaine of Maine, and Grover Cleveland of New York. Herr Lanfer and Josef agreed they were concerned about having a Democrat president if Cleveland was to win, as it would be the first Democrat president since the war between the states. Alfred felt it would be a welcome addition and shake up the White House. It all ended well as Mrs. Lanfer said, "Ihr Männer fängt besser an zu essen und hört auf zu reden! "

Now I knew a bit of German, but I was lost.

Josef could see in my expression, "Alice, she said you men better start eating and quit yakking so much."

We all laughed.

After dinner, we went to the main room and played cards. It was so much fun; we laughed most of the night. I felt relaxed with this very loving family.

Since it was so dark outside, Johanna's mother recommended that Alfred and Josef would take me home in their buggy. Johanna came too, and we both sat in the back of the buggy, chatting the whole way.

As we got home Josef helped me off the buggy and escorted me up to the door of my home. *Such a gentleman*, I thought.

I went to bed that night, wondering if I would meet Josef again. If there was such a thing as love at first sight, I thought this might be it.

But as the days passed, I never heard from him. I realized this love might only be one way. Johanna and I never discussed him, either.

Very soon after, I took on the role of Maw's #1 assistant, as Beu was cutting back even more on the births she attended. She told Maw she would do more of the chores at home and tend to the animals. Maw frequently sent me out to sit with women and prepare their homes for birthing. I even caught a few babies before she arrived. I usually took care of the healthy mamas.

I really do not feel ready to help women birth on my own. But hold on there, wait a minute, I thought.

*I **am** helping women birth on my own. At least five times so far.*

If Maw was unsure of the home, or we attended a birth at a brothel, we would always go together. She always stressed the importance of *letting birth happen.* To encourage women to move and respond to their babies.

Additionally, she stressed the importance of *not* having women push before they were ready. You should wait for her to have the urge to push. Better yet, could you see the head — or even just hair? It was vital to wait for the head to emerge and rotate.
If a midwife instructed a mother to push too soon, undue swelling could occur, which could block the birth canal and prevent the baby from descending.

It was also very important to let the placenta's blood drain into the baby before cutting the cord.

All this advice was helpful when the birth was typical.

But births weren't always typical.

One night, I was sent out ahead to help a young woman birth her second baby. Albert had come to our home to deliver the message. He offered to drive me in, as it was late, and I accepted. Maw told me she would meet up with me later. I grabbed the big bag to take with me.

As we took the buggy to town, I realized I had never been to this side of Milwaukee. I asked Albert, "Who are these men having their horses pull large carts with barrels through the city? I have seen at least seven carts go by?"

"Oh, these are the *night soil men*. While the city sleeps under the cloak of darkness, these brave men empty the latrines and cesspools of human waste. So, our proper folk don't have to bear the burden of witnessing their excrement be hauled away during the daytime hours." [H-1]

We soon arrived. Albert said he would go back to check on Maw and see if she was ready to come. Then would return in the morning.

Albert told me more about this couple. The young woman, Maggie, had moved out west with her husband, Luke. Luke worked in a new steel factory in Milwaukee. Maggie's mother had come to town to help her, but sadly she had to leave back to their home in Ohio, as Maggie's father had fallen ill.

Luke and Maggie lived in a small flat on the west side. The steel mill company owned the building and rented the apartments out to the men and their families.

I grabbed my bag and walked up the steps to their apartment. I knocked on the door, and an older lady answered. She was holding a young girl in her arms, perhaps two or three years old.

I inquired, "Is this the home of Luke and Maggie Johnson?"

"It sure is you must be Clara," said the lady.

"No, I am her daughter Alice. Clara will be coming later."

"Well, I am Andrea, I live in the flat below. There is Maggie sitting on the couch."

"Hi Maggie, I am Alice. How are you?"

"In labor, I am sure of it. My pains are every five minutes. And my little girl Sofiia is in Andrea's arms. She has been getting upset every time my labor pains come. We can see how long she will last."

Andrea said, "If this is too much for Sofiia, I can take her down to my flat. Maggie's husband Luke should be here soon."

"Oh, here it comes! Whew — whew — whew. Oh no. Whew — whew — whew. Wow, this was a big one."

Sofiia started to cry in the background. "Mommy. I want my Mommy!"

Andrea comforted her, and after exchanging a look with Maggie, excused herself to take Sofia to her apartment.

Maggie was happy to have me there. This was her second birth, so I thought it might go a bit quicker. I carefully washed my hands and elbows with soap. I brought some knitting to do, just in case.

Several hours passed, and Luke still had yet to arrive. Maggie reassured me he would come.

The labor was gradually progressing.

Maggie continued to move around the room, all in an effort to get comfortable. Yet, she never seemed to feel comfortable.

Several more hours passed, but everything was going well with the labor — until her water broke.

It was tainted with dark green muck. I had not seen this before.

When I looked more closely, I noticed her belly was misshapen.

"I know you want Luke here, Maggie, but I believe you will be birthing soon."

"Oh, Alice, I might as well tell you. Luke is in jail. I think he will be out real soon." Maggie scuffled to talk as she was looking distressed. "He's in jail for a crime he didn't commit — well, kind of. Sort of. Andrea's husband is going to town to talk with the Sheriff to see if he can get Luke out."

"Here it is again — whew, whew, whew — and another - whew- whew. This is too much; I can't take this. Is something wrong? Much more painful than my last birth." Sweat was dripping off her forehead.

I rarely checked the woman unless the birth was not progressing as expected. This was one of those births.

I reached in my hand and did not feel a hard head or hair. I felt a spongy soft part. My finger slipped into a hole, and as I withdrew, I noticed more black, tarry, sticky muck on my finger.

What is this? The baby's feces? Where was Maw?

I was scared but remained composed.

I had helped women birth before. What was going on? I tried to recall anything that would help.

I remember once doing a vaginal inspection on a woman who was not progressing. I felt a hole and could feel the baby sucking on my finger. It was the baby's mouth. Maw told me that the baby was face up. For starters, we made that mother lay over the bed with her knees up. We ended up turning that mama and baby in all kinds of positions. Getting the baby in the right position was so important, so its neck wouldn't be hurt.

Still, Maggie's birth was different.

I thought. *Since this was indeed not the head, it must be the baby's bottom.* [B-7]

Yes, of course, soft and spongy, plus the tarry feces that most babies have.

"Alice, it's coming. I have the urge. Ahhhhh." Maggie began to start shaking, barely able to withstand the pain.

Maggie wanted to push. The baby's bottom did expel…a bit later, one leg of the baby at a time dropped down. Then came the baby's belly, cord and all.

Oh no! Not the cord, I thought.

If the cord came out now, it could get stuck and stop pulsating. I could feel it on the baby's abdomen; it felt deflated, and I could feel the cord's beats. They were slowing down.

The cord was getting stuck.

"Maggie," I said. "Don't push hard; just gentle blows."

"Okay. Okay. I will. Whew — whew...what's happening?" cried out Maggie.

The baby's right shoulder popped out. I grabbed the right elbow and out came the arm. Now it was easier for the left side to expel.
Everything but the head had been expelled, and the hanging body was motionless just as Maw walked in. She could see what was happening and the *terror* in my eyes.

She walked over to help me, "Alice, let the baby hang down for a minute."

I did.

It seemed like forever.

Maw and I changed places. Then, I saw Maw struggle to reach in the birth opening with one hand. She was able to get in. Later, I found out she placed her finger in the baby's mouth and pulled the chin down to flex. She grabbed the baby's ankles and pulled up with her other hand.[B-7]

"Alice, grab that towel over there." She pointed to the chair. "I will give you the baby. I want you to vigorously rub the baby until it breathes before placing it on Maggie's chest."

The baby was born — blue as can be — and went straight into my arms. I dried and roused the baby. The baby remained blue and floppy. I continued to rub the baby's back. "Come on baby, breathe — baby, breathe. You can do it, little one," I whispered to the baby.

"What's going on? Will my baby be okay? Oh no. Please, God!" cried out Maggie.

I continued to rub and dry. Nothing was happening.

"You're doing good Alice. Keep it up," said Maw.

I began to worry. But then, something happened. Gradually, the baby started to pink up, and I noticed the cord starting to plump. As I rubbed the baby's back, I could hear its gurgling turn into a deep breath.

Soon we heard a big cry! Everyone in the room smiled! We welcomed that incessant crying.

I felt like I was missing something.

Oh yeah — the announcement.

I looked at Maggie. "Maggie, it's a girl!" I placed the crying baby on her chest.

Soon, the I felt the cord stop pulsating. Maw handed me the string and knife; I created two ties close to the baby's belly. Then, I made the cut.

Soon after, a gush of blood was expelled from Maggie, and the remaining cord lengthened. I knew the placenta would be next.

Next, the placenta was expelled, and Maw gently massaged Maggie's uterus until it became firm and reduced in size to just below her belly button.
A few hours later, we heard a knock on the door. I answered it.

It was Andrea's husband, with a note in his hand. "This is for Maggie," he said, nodding at her before leaving.

I handed the note to Maggie. As soon as she read it, she started to cry.

"We are here for you, Maggie. Is everything okay?" I said.

"It's from the Sheriff," sniveled Maggie, holding up the note to read it to us. "Mrs. Johnson, we regret to inform you that your husband, Luke, will remain in jail until a trial can be held. He cannot be released any sooner." ... She looked up at us. "This doesn't seem right. How am I going to manage everything?"

"Time is a great healer; let's see what happens," I said.

Just then, Andrea returned to the apartment. "Sofia fell asleep on our couch. She seemed exhausted. My husband will come to get us if he needs us. Alice and Clara, I can take it from here."

"Andrea, thanks so much," I said. "Please watch Maggie and the baby closely. Come here, and I will show you how to massage the uterus." I then instructed her how to massage and gave her supplies to care for them. We hugged Maggie and were glad she had already started to breastfeed.

By then, it was early morning. Maw and I left; we walked down the stairs to meet up with Albert. To our pleasant surprise, he was outside waiting for us.

As we drove home, I reflected on this birth that had been full of surprises. I was lucky. I was scared. I was thankful. This birth happened, albeit mostly on its own.

I guess I could say I knew what I was doing.

Well. Not exactly.

I successfully managed myself while attending to this complicated birth. I was relieved and beaming with joy at the same time.

Now, Maggie and Luke were the parents of a beautiful baby girl, and Sofia was a big sister. My only concern at this point was whether Luke would be released. What had he done?

As I learned how to assist women with birth, I was told vaginal inspections were rarely done, as we didn't want to cause a fever. Grandma had told me horror stories of people placing their dirty hands in there and leaving mothers with filthy diseases. Yet at times, I knew they were needed.

Maggie's abdomen appeared to be misshapen. My gut had told me something was wrong. Was it correct to do a vaginal inspection? I thought it was. In this case, the baby's hole in her bottom helped identify what part of her body was coming.

I asked Maw about letting the baby hang. This did not make sense to me at the time. She explained that this birth was considered *breech* since it was not the head coming out first. With this type of bottom-first birth, you could injure the woman's birth canal or the baby's neck if you weren't careful. By letting the baby hang, the baby's head would flex chin-to-chest, and the weight of the dangling baby would place pressure on the baby's head to emerge. If letting the baby hang didn't work, you could reach up, flex the head, and pull up the legs before the baby could descend. Maw had done this before.

All of these strategies could help ensure a healthy birth for mama and baby.

I sat back and smiled for the whole rest of the home.

I was excited to have another tool in my midwife toolbox. Now I could help even more mothers and their babies.

Susan E. Fleming

Alice Ada Wood: Midwife Apprentice

CHAPTER 6
EDUCATING THE MIDWEST: BIRTHING & NURSING
MILWAUKEE - 1885

In 1885, our family moved from the countryside of Milwaukee to Wauwatosa Town. Wauwatosa is Pottawatomie Indian name for "firefly." It was named after the fireflies that would light a path alongside the river at night.

Pa said this part of town was up-and-coming since the train tracks went right through the town. Very large homes were being built, which meant lots of work for Pa. He also especially liked being next to the Menomonee River to go fishing. Maw felt safer for her family here, away from the big city. Grandma

French came with us too. She was still complaining about that *darn wobbling frying pan.* Pa would always roll his eyes when she did.

I was still in high school and would have to find another one to attend. The nursing school was coming to town in three or four years. Maw and Grandma were still determined to see me go there. I still wasn't sure what I felt about it — so often, school never seemed to teach what I really needed to learn.

I was also saddened to leave my school friend Johanna. We agreed to keep in touch, as we still didn't live far from each other.

One afternoon, Maw and Grandma traveled to Milwaukee to hear a presentation at the hospital. There, heard doctors talk about the upcoming establishment of education for nurses and doctors in Milwaukee.

I only found out after they came home.

That night at dinner, Grandma urged my mother, "Clara, tell the family what we learned today."

Maw said, "Grandma, I don't think they are interested. Maybe Alice."

"Maybe next time you can take me," I said.

Maw smiled at the frustration in my tone. She knew I thought normal high school wasn't serving my needs.

"We didn't want to take you out of school. Besides, we can tell you now. If it's not too much for everyone else." She looked at her son.

Eddie was dozing.

Pa gave him a shove. "We are interested too. Aren't we, son?"

Eddie startled and nodded. "Why sure, Pops!"

Everyone in the house listened attentively as Maw reported on the day.

"Grandma and I attended a presentation at the Passavant Hospital in Milwaukee. There were many businessmen and men from the railroads there, and the goal of the hospital was to increase funding for our new nursing school. A visiting doctor named Neil Shaw from New York City gave the talk. He supported an apprentice model to train the nurses and doctors in the Midwest until we could expand our colleges and Universities in America. Milwaukee will be part of the change. The Milwaukee County Training School of Nursing will be established very soon. It will be a start!"

"Good to hear, Clara. Sounds like Milwaukee has a vested interest in bringing medical education right here in our community. Those railroad men will be big contributors to the nursing school, as they want Milwaukee to thrive as they increase the number of transcontinental railroads," said Pa.

I was not as thrilled as Pa and Maw seemed to be. Who needed school when you could learn on the job?

Later that evening, I met with Pa, Maw, and Grandma in the gathering room. They expressed confidence in me, as I had done well in my new high school.

"With grades like you have, Alice, you will be welcomed as a student for the new nursing school," stated Pa.

On one hand, I was flattered that they believed in me, but on the other hand, I was not quite sure if the nursing school was what I wanted to do.

Besides, I wasn't so sure about hospitals. Maw's war stories made them seem like disgusting, despairing places. A hospital seems so cold. And I had heard from one of my friends at school who went to a hospital in Chicago that they stunk. I really did not want to be in one of those smelly hospitals.

One week later, Maw and Grandma finally invited me to join them to listen to a nurse from Scotland who would be visiting the Saint Mary's Hospital in Milwaukee. The local doctors and the hospital staff recommended that all community nurses, midwives, and birth attendants attend next Friday afternoon. Beu expressed no interest.

I was somewhat excited to go. I was interested in learning more about midwifery. But why was a nurse from Scotland coming here? What did she know that we didn't?

That Friday afternoon, we dressed up in our finest attire. I put on my long dark blue skirt and favorite cream-colored blouse.

Pa pulled up with the buggy in front of the house. As we walked down, I saw that Pa had dressed as a coachman wearing his best attire: a box coat with a top hat. He escorted all three of us to the Saint Mary's Hospital in Milwaukee. During the lecture, he tended horses and visited local shops.

He dropped us out in front of the hospital as he offered his hand to help each of us to step off the buggy.

We entered the hospital and asked the front desk where to go. They directed us down to the Fredrick and Gretchen Schultz Lecture Hall. We made our way down there and sat just in time for the event.

Miss Caroline Hollinsworth introduced herself.[B-9, H-3] She was certified as a nurse from the City of Edinburgh's General Lying-In Hospital. We had read from the flyer that she was a nursing instructor ten years ago and was part of a panel investigating Florence Nightingale's writings in her pioneer study on maternal mortality, *Introductory Notes on Lying-in Institutions*. Today, Miss Hollinsworth was part of a research team from London working to reduce maternal deaths throughout the United Kingdom. She was excited to be invited to travel to this part of the New World.

She stated: "One of the most dangerous complications of birthing on our island is *haemorrrhage*.[B-10, H-3] Defined by its copious amounts of bleeding; this condition is known to raise anxiety in nearly every attendant." Many of the midwives and nurses in the audience nodded their heads. "If the haemorrrhage starts at the middle to the end of pregnancy, this is known as *placenta praevia*,[B-11] whereas haemorrrhage that happens after the birth is known as *post-partal*."H-3

She asked the audience, "How many of you have heard of *placenta praevia?*" Only a few raised their hands. She continued, "Only the Good Lord in Heaven knows why a few women experience a placenta that comes first. You often see this in women who are experiencing bright red bleeding during the mid – late part of their pregnancy."

"In London, we have an obstetrician named Braxton Hicks who is working on this. Right now, the treatment of caring for a woman with placental praevia is a complicated procedure that should only be done in the confines of a hospital. With your primitive healthcare system here in America, professional physicians and midwives might not be available. I highly recommend the following treatments to do in the homes."

She looked around. "I'm having a flyer passed around with treatment advice for placenta praevia.[11] Please keep and consult — and pass the knowledge on to your friends who couldn't be here."

Haemorrrhage Treatments for Home Care[H-3]
Miss Caroline Hollingsworth

Treatment for placenta praevia[B-11]:
- First, upon inspection, you may notice a lumpy presenting part. Leave it alone unless there is copious bleeding. Then possibly, try packing.
- Try to Transfer to a hospital — as many hands may save lives.
- If bleeding is severe, consider it an eminent crisis that can result in the death of the baby as well as the mother. Time is not your friend. Do your best.

Treatment for post-partal haemorrrhage[B-10]:
- Rub and knead the uterus.
- Give a drachm of Ergot in a wine glass of hot water. Preferably after the placenta is delivered.

After everyone had received their flyer, she waited a moment to make sure they were read before continuing.

"Let me share a verse for you to consider remembering when treating an emergent case.

> *If the Face is Red - Raise the Head.*
> *If the Face is Pale - Raise the Tale.*

Do you have any questions?"

A midwife in the audience asked, "Why do you prefer to give the ergot after the placenta is delivered?"

I was also curious. Some people say Ergot could stop bleeding and help pain in the correct doses.

Miss Hollinsworth nodded. "From my personal experience of watching ergot administered before the placenta is delivered, I have seen placental entrapment, resulting in the death of the woman. Even if you give it after, please be cautious with giving too much ergot, as it can result in your mother having fits. This too can result in death."

After a round of questions, she continued her talk. I admired her confidence as she spoke.

"Now I would like to discuss child-bed fever, also known as *puerperal fever*. Every maternal death from puerperal fever is a disgrace to civilization."

Miss Hollinsworth then shared the Semmelweis story.

Ignatz Semmelweis and doctors' hygiene [B-12, H-3]

In 1846, Ignatz Semmelweis, a young intern in the obstetric clinic in Vienna, Austria, noticed that the local midwives' clinic had a 1.5 percent mortality rate, whereas the medical students' clinic had a 15 percent mortality rate. The midwives taunted the medical students about the disparity.

Then, one of Semmelweis's colleagues contracted disease in his finger during a postmortem. He succumbed to sepsis. Semmelweis was outraged at the neglect of cleanliness. He realized that medical students were attending autopsies in the morgue and then traveling straight to the confinement room of women ready to birth.

Immediately, he required that students wash their hands with chlorine water after the autopsies and before attending to the pregnant women. Miraculously, mortality rate at the medical students' obstetric clinic plummeted below that of the midwives' clinic.

"I cannot stress this enough. Every woman in the room caring for pregnant women must learn about hygiene — even, as in the case of Semmelweis, just washing your hands. Are any of you taking hygienic precautions as you care for women during exams or births?"

Very few women in the group raised their hands. Maw was one of them.

Miss Hollinsworth pointed to her. "Tell us what you do."

Maw shared with the group. "With our births, we scrub our hands to our elbows several times during a birth — just as we enter the home, then again right before inspection, and any time we soil our hands. Finally, we do it one last time before we leave the home."

Miss Hollinsworth said, "Brilliant! That is quite forward-thinking care. Where did you acquire this information from?"

"I base our hand hygiene etiquette on my work as a nurse in a field hospital during the war between the states."

"Tell us, what antiseptic do you use?"

"Normally, we use salve that we make with animal fat and lye. We may sprinkle carbolic acid on the floor to reduce the stench. If the woman or place is really dirty, we also use carbolic acid as an antiseptic. It is painful and tough on the skin but controls gangrene. We used it in the war to clean out wounds. After washing our hands, we make sure to rinse them immediately. My mother has created a salve to soften our skin."

Miss Hollinsworth replied, "Homemade salves are helpful. You might also consider using an iodine tincture as an antiseptic rather than carbolic acid when tending to your very sick folks. Check with your chemist at your local medicine stores to get some."

She continued. "I understand that here in Milwaukee, as well as other parts of the United States, nearly all the births are conducted in the homes — and that most of you have no formal midwifery training like we are proposing in many parts of the United Kingdom. Formal training would typically be three to six months for those trained as nurses."

"I don't want to forget to tell you. When caring for an ill mother, I highly recommend keeping all opium away from infants. Ingesting opium could be devastating for a baby."

She ended with a sentiment I would think a lot about. "I was also just made aware that maternal childcare will not be in the upcoming nursing program. I find that quite disappointing. I highly encourage you to be involved with the program."

A social followed the presentation, where tea and crumpets were served. It was wonderful to meet our guests from Great Britain and other midwives and nurses in our community.

I approached the speaker. "Miss Hollingsworth, may I speak with you?"

"Of course. Your name?"

"My name is Alice Wood; I am a midwife apprentice here in town. We were surprised to hear that the nursing school would not include maternity childcare. You suggested we should be involved. What do you recommend?"

Miss Hollingsworth smiled. "Well, of course. After a nursing school is established in Milwaukee, please attend and inspire medical professionals to consider a form of midwifery training alongside the nursing program."

She then leaned in and whispered. "Your men in this community are quite highhanded. That is why I recommend you inspire them *after* attending school." She winked.

That made more sense. I smiled. "Thank you for taking the time to speak with us."

"Why, of course. Is that lady over there your mother?"

"Yes, she is."

"Quite a bright woman, she is."

"We think so too."

We met Pa and took our buggy home, inspired by Miss Hollinsworth. We decided to go see our local chemist Mr. Akers and see if we could add more ergot and opium and, of course, a better antiseptic to our midwifery supplies. Grandma and I praised Maw for speaking up and sharing her talent. I was grateful to be part of our family birthing group.

Susan E. Fleming

CHAPTER 7
EXPERIENCING VIOLENCE:
SINS OF THE LAWLESS - 1885

Even after we moved to Wauwatosa Town, Eddie and I still had a long walk of over three miles to school.

It was much further than before — but it was considerably more beautiful since we could walk along the river. Our new school was close to the town, next to a hardware store.

It was June, and the last day of school for the year had just ended. Eddie and I were walking home. The summer flowers were covering the hills, and tree line forest bordered our walking path.

Suddenly, I remembered that I had left my favorite notebook at school. I did want it for the summer break.

I told Eddie, "Go ahead and go home. I will meet up with you later."

He gladly agreed since he wanted to meet Pa and go fishing.

I was almost to the school when I saw a man sitting on a fence along the side of the road — a stranger. He reminded me of Annabelle's' brother.

He was a large man who was unkempt and unshaven. As I approached, he gave me a horrific look. I felt like he looked at me as if I had no clothes on as he gazed over my body. I wore a nice full skirt and a buttoned-up jacket, but it didn't help.

I tried to pass him as quickly as possible, but he spoke, and I stopped. "Hello, pretty lady, can you tell me where the hardware store is?"

I pointed up the road. "You can find it just up the road next to the school." I swiftly walked away.

Soon, I heard him walking behind me as I got closer to the school. His footsteps sounded louder as he got closer.

Then, the footsteps disappeared.

Thank goodness; what a relief.

I was so happy to get away from him. I quickly walked to the school's front door; I would get help from our teacher.

But the door was locked.

Since it was the last day, our teacher must have left early.

I considered my options.

I could go to the hardware store, but what if that man was there? That would be horrible.

I decided I just wanted to get home.

Fast.

The road was quiet on the way back. There was a stillness in the air. I didn't hear any birds singing. I was about halfway home, and then. There he was, in front of me.

I could feel myself starting to tremble. I knew this was not going to be a good encounter.

He approached me. "Hello again, beautiful."

I didn't meet his eyes. "Please excuse me. I need to get home fast and feed our animals." I tried to walk past him.

Then it happened.

He grabbed me and threw me to the side of the road near the forest.

I immediately tried to stand, but he was on me.

He pushed me down again.

I was horrified. I managed to stand up and tried to hit him.

He grabbed my wrist.

My mind was racing.

What can I do? I thought. *How can I get away from this tyrant?*

I started to scream, but he placed his hand over my mouth. My screams were muffled. *Who would hear me?*

He punched me in the face — and then it was hard to think much of anything.

He sat on me and pulled a scarf out of his pocket. *He's gonna stuff it in my mouth,* I realized.

And he did.

Then he tied the rest of it through my mouth and behind my head.

I scratched his face and kicked him as much as I could. It didn't have any effect. This large and brutal man knew what he was doing.

I teared up and closed my eyes as he started kissing and licking my face. I felt like retching.

At this point, I knew there was no way out. I could not push him away or fight him off.

He laid on me, making the most repulsive moves, pressing his privates against mine.

I tried locking my ankles together with my ankles. Surely, he could not break my locked legs.

He did.

He took off his pants, and he was on me again. He pushed my skirt up and ripped my jacket open. The buttons went flying. He grabbed my breast with one hand as he shoved his man part inside me. This became quite painful. I found it hard to withstand. My eyes tear. My whole body felt numb.

He did it.

He kept at it, all while making animal sounds. It was nauseating to hear him.

Will I survive? I thought. *Is he going to kill me?*

My heart was racing. I felt myself trying to crawl out

of my body and escape.

Suddenly, I heard a loud *thud*, and a huge weight fell on me. I was being smothered.

I felt something warm and wet and copper-smelling coming down over my eyes, face, and neck.

Blood.

Was this it? Was I going to die? Did he just shoot me? What was happening?

He was slumped over me. He didn't move.

Like he was lifeless.

For a moment, I thought he was dead.

I heard faint sounds. I almost thought I could hear my grandmother. Oh, how I loved her.

Then, I realized — *I do hear my grandmother.*

"Alice, is that you?"

My Grandmother French stood holding up her new

frying pan from the hardware store.

"Grandma!"

She dropped the pan, almost weeping, and grabbed the man.

"Help me push that tormentor off you, girl."

So, I did. I pushed, with all my strength. He was unconscious and slumped off me. His head was bloody.

I struggled to sit up. Grandma fell on me, untying my mouth, and helping me up.

"Hurry," she said, as I stood. "Let's get out of here before he wakes up."

I arranged my clothes the best I could, and we got out of there.

We were both walking so fast, we were nearly running home.

Not a word was said.
As we entered the house, there sat everyone at the

dinner table.

Maw looked horrified at the sight of me.

I collapsed on the couch, unable to move. Pa and Eddie were stunned and speechless. Beulah started to cry. Grandma quickly sat in her comfy chair.

Still, not a word was said.

Obviously, *something* had happened to me. Blood was still dripping off my face. My clothes, my jacket, and skirt were torn, and the buttons ripped off. My arms and legs were bruised, and my left eye was blackened.

Maw came over and sat by me on the couch.

She broke the silence. "Ok family — something terrible has happened to Alice and Grandma. Grandma French, tell us what happened."

"I will, Clara," Grandma said. "Let me catch my breath!"

You could see her trying to compose herself. "I had taken a buggy ride to the hardware store to buy that new frying pan. I was hoping to meet up with Alice and Eddie at the school. I went to the school and saw that the door was locked. Little Johnny Danklefsen came up to me and told me that the school had closed early and that he had just seen Alice running home on the trail. I wasn't sure if I could catch up with her. But I did decide to walk on home anyway rather than hire a carriage ride. I had just past the Menomonee River, and I was heading by the forest when I heard rustling in the woods of a man and a woman. I tried not to look, but I could tell the woman was trying to fight against the man. Then, I recognized Alice's skirt, which was nearly ripped off. I don't know what got into me. But the next thing I remembered, there laid a man unconscious with blood squirting out of his head."

She took another breath. "I think I might have hit him in the head with my new frying pan. I called for Alice to help me move him off her. I quickly grabbed the man's knife and slashed the scarf that was in Alice's mouth. I then threw his knife into the woods…he won't be needing that anymore. I helped her up, and we ran home as quickly as possible."

Grandma fought some emotion in her voice. "I was too late ..."

As I lay on the couch, I could hear every word that was said.

What did Grandma mean that she was too late? *Was I ruined for life?*

Maw said we could report to the police, but then everyone in town would know what happened since the newspapers always publish the victim's name and who did the crime. So horrible. I would not want that!

I could hear Maw and Pa quarreling. I didn't care to follow what they were saying.

Eddie came by my side. "Sis, I am so sorry. I should have walked back to the school with you."

I could see he was tearing up. It made me gather my strength and sit up. I gave him a big hug and reassured him. "Eddie, none of us knew this would happen. Don't fret."

"Eddie?" Pa said. He had his and Eddie's gun.

Eddie nodded yet he stood still.

Pa grabbed him as they headed out the door.

And we ladies started to talk about what to do next.

Grandma asked, "Alice, when was your last bleed?"

I told her, "It just ended on Monday."

She nodded. "Well then, most likely, you will not be pregnant."

"Mother, that is an old wives' tale," Maw said.

We all decided to wait and see. I was so scared.

Beu asked, "Can I get you some water to drink?"

I nodded yes.

Meanwhile, Grandma and Maw prepared a vinegar wash to cleanse me. They also warmed up some water on the stove to allow me to relax in an Epsom salt bath.

After cleaning up and taking a bath. Maw offered to

make me a bed on the couch. I told her I just wanted to go up to my own bed. She helped me up the ladder to sleep in the loft. We talked a bit more as I laid down.

"I know I took a bath, but I still feel dirty. Like I can't get clean. I am worried that everyone will know what happened."

"You are terrified, Alice. This is expected. You need time to recuperate. Stay home for at least a few weeks. Maybe more. I will bring in Charlene to help with midwifing for a while. You'll need to care for yourself before you can care for others."

She gave me a big hug as she left. I laid in bed thinking. *Would a man like Josef would ever call on a woman like me? Was it too late?*

There was one saving grace — I had a mother and grandmother who were not only willing to talk to me about this but also insisted that we needed to talk. It was so helpful.

With time, I did calm down.

I later found out that Pa and Eddie rode into town.

They gathered some men from Pa's work and looked for the man. They found him at a bar drinking. His face was scratched up.
That is all that I ever heard. I never ever found out what happened.

Violence in the untamed midwest was not only prevalent, it was seething.

No one seemed accountable.

Susan E. Fleming

CHAPTER 8
BIRTHING-TOO-SOON:
MULTIPLES, DISEASES, OR VIOLENCE?
MILWAUKEE 1886

By 1886, I was 18 years of age.

It took time for me to decide to go back to birthing.

Maw and I had a long discussion about my sorrow and my future in midwifing.

I soon realized I was not the only one on this earth suffering. While I cared for others, I recognized that so many people are suffering — many, much more than I.

And I could help.

So, I decided to go back to working with Maw.

I had a new outlook on my life. I was grateful to have found my calling, which was to help women with birthing.

Women need us.

On occasion, Maw and I were called to assist a woman whose pregnancy was ending too soon. Usually, we did not meet mamas until a few weeks before they were to give birth — or even just on birthing day.

With babies born early, it was usually different. Typically, a mama would have cramping, discharge, or bleeding. This would cause an alarm. Maw said that in cases of early birth, we must consider multiples (two or more babies), violence, or diseases such as syphilis, even in the most religious homes.

Emma was one of those moms.

Maw suggested we take our horses since we had to travel four or five miles out of town. Emma lived on a small farm, away from other homes close by. She was twenty-four years old and requested that Maw and I come to her home.

As we entered her home, we noticed she was very quiet. Maw decided to first take time to get to know her. I sat on the floor to play blocks with her children so that Emma could talk better with Maw. We both noticed that with time, she began to relax.

She told us a bit about herself. She had only been married four years, and her husband was quite a bit older — he was forty-seven years old, to be exact. Her husband was gone on a hunting expedition. She was home caring for her two young children, ages nine months and two and one-half years old. Her last two pregnancies were uneventful.

We found out that Emma and her husband were heading west. They had met in Boston. However, when their funds became tight, they decided to stop in Milwaukee, as her husband could work at the local mill. She had three sisters back home.

Maw asked her, "What made you decide to have us come here today?"

Emma responded, "I noticed I am discharging some dark blood."[B-13]

Maw frowned. "That's concerning. May we check you?"

Emma nodded.

Maw instructed, "Lie down here on the couch while I listen to your baby."

Emma lay down.

Maw pulled out her wooden Pinard horn to listen to Emma's baby. The horn was a gift from Maw's grandmother, Grandma French's mother, Mary Ferris, when Grandma left New York.

Maw confirmed that she heard the baby. She also noticed that Emma had a bruise on her lower abdomen and that her abdomen was quite tight, almost rigid. [B-13]

Maw probed. "Are you feeling the baby move at all?"

"I can feel the baby move, but maybe not as often," Emma admitted.

At times we must ask hard questions, but it helps us decide how to move forward. However, we don't always get the truth.

Maw told Emma that she noticed a bruise on her abdomen. "Has anyone hit you recently?"

Emma answered quickly — too quickly.

"Oh, I did not know I had a bruise. It must have come when I slipped outside feeding the animals. I didn't think much about that."

Maw then inquired, "Is your husband helpful?"

Emma confirmed, "Of course he is. He is very good at providing us a home and money for food."

Maw's mouth was tight. She didn't believe her.

Finally, Maw said, "Okay. I know it's hard with young ones but try to rest on the couch. Let us know if anything changes, such as more contractions or bleeding." She stood. "You may recall something

you forgot to tell us. I will see if I can send ladies from the church to help you with meals and watch the children while your husband is gone."
Maw made to leave. I followed.

Emma called out.

"Clara, before you leave — I believe you know my Mama. She worked with you in the hospital near Gettysburg during the War. Her name is Abigail. Abi is from South Carolina. She told me to contact you."

Maw smiled. "Of course, I know Abi; we worked in the field hospital together. We not only saved many legs, but we also saved lives! She lived in our home for over a year. Will you send her my best?"

"I will be happy to do that. Thanks again for your help."

We left.

On our ride home, Maw shared more about Abi.

"Abi was a lovely nurse, dear friend, and a sister in the gospel. Just before the war broke out, a slave owner and old friend of my father traveled north and stayed at our inn in New York during the late autumn of 1860. He brought a slave girl with him, which was not uncommon. He met with my father and asked if he could leave her here in our home before he traveled back to his home in South Carolina since he feared the war would break out soon. My father asked him how well did he know this girl? He confided to my father that his own wife was barren and that he had relations with one of his slaves, and this was *his daughter*. This slave girl was Abi. He wanted her to be free.

He also told my father that she was well-versed in assisting with birthing and nursing.

Abi stayed with us for a year. After she moved out, she found a wonderful man at church named Spencer. Soon they were married. We all felt the war was coming, and it did! Spencer left for the war. Spencer did not know that Abi was pregnant with their first child. This child was Emma.

Sadly, in 1862, Spencer was killed in a bloody battle in Maryland at a place called Antietam Creek.

To our surprise, the war went on for a few more years. When we saw the war was escalating, the Union had a draft. My dad had lost my brother, his only son, but was determined to help the cause. He sent two of my sisters and me to the front lines of the War to help as nurses."[B-14.]

"Maw, that was quite bold for Grandfather to send his family to the front lines of a major war."

"You must understand, Alice, that we, too, wanted to help. At that time, we were all worried the war would come to us - in our homes and farms in western New York. That is what had happened in the French Indian war... My sisters and I went to serve as nurses. This is when Abi decided to join us as a nurse to work at one of the field hospitals near Gettysburg in Pennsylvania. The hospital was set up in a church."

"What an amazing story! So, Maw, is Abi mulattoe?"

"Yes, she is. That is what made her so beautiful," declared Maw.

"What about Emma?"

"Emma is what we call *passing,* which means passing as a white person," acknowledged Maw. "Alice many people heading west are passing. Maybe even a few in our family lines."

As we continued to travel, I sensed that Maw felt we didn't get the whole story. So, as we traveled down the road on our horses, I asked her to share her thoughts.

Maw shared, "Alice, most of the time, I believe what my mothers tell me. This was not one of those times. My gut says she is not telling the truth. First, the bruise was low on her abdomen. Right by her pubic bone. Typically, when you fall, you hit the part that is sticking out the most. When I see dark blood, I think of old blood. I have seen this on a woman who fell off her buggy before. She lost her baby a week later. I have also seen this when a husband kicks the mama. It typically is on the lower abdomen. Just like Emma.[B-13] The baby's heart rate was low, which alone is concerning."

I agreed with Maw; it just didn't seem right. She confirmed that we could only hope Emma recovered or called us back to help.

A month later, Emma called us back. We went inside her home, and she started to cry. She wanted to tell us what was happening. "I am so ashamed. I birthed the baby two weeks ago. It was a little boy. He was stillborn. I buried him in my backyard by my favorite oak tree."

She had only been six months pregnant.

Now for the truth: "I didn't slip tending to the animals. Just before my husband left, we got into a fight. I suspected my husband was going to the local brothels, as he would come home late with lipstick on his shirt. He was unhappy that the first two babies were so close but became livid to find out I was pregnant again. That is when he kicked me in the abdomen."

What a horrible man, I thought. *Emma deserves better.*

We could see that Emma was recovering well. At least, her body was. Her belly was soft, and her uterus was below her pelvis bone. She had been feeding her nine-month-old baby, so she had milk.

Maw suggested that Emma contact her family to help. Or Maw could even send a telegram to Abi or her sisters.

Emma said, "Great idea. I will contact my mother and my three sisters. I am sure they can send me money to come home to Boston. We can take a train."

Maw offered, "Sounds like a good plan, Emma. We can come by with our buggy to get you and the girls to the train headed east."

She agreed. We helped Emma clean up her house and then left.

But we never heard from her.

I guessed I needed to be grateful she had called upon us earlier at all. Boston will be a better place for her to raise her children. She needed her family.

As we rode home on our horses, Maw told me yet another story, which took place back in New York around the time just before the war.

"A group of recent woman immigrants from France called themselves Basques. Many of their husbands were sheepherders, while the women worked at bakeries. One thing quite a few of these ladies had in common was that they would have their first pregnancy without incident. Nevertheless, subsequent pregnancies often ended in early deliveries, usually resulting in the baby's death.[B-15] The lead woman came to my grandma for help. Grandma and I felt helpless," Maw accounted.

"What was happening, Maw; was it a bad illness?"

"We never found out. Neither of us had experienced caring for ladies with these types of pregnancy complications."

What could have been happening to these women? [B-15]

One afternoon, I was resting on the porch taking in the heat.

It was a warm summer day. The warm rain started to fall on the roof. Surprisingly, I saw a young man riding up to our house.

It was Josef.

What was he doing here?

From his horse, he asked, "May I join you, Alice?" "Why of course. Please take a seat up here on the porch."

He stepped down from his horse and tied him to a post. He came to the porch and sat on the chair beside mine.

The summer storm raged. The rain pinged on the roof. We heard every drop. A coolness tinged the air.

I looked at him and smiled. He smiled back.

Once the rain subsided, Josef asked, "Would you like to walk with me?"

I was thrilled.

Trying not to act too excited, I said, "That would be nice, Josef. Let me tell my family that I am leaving."

I opened the front door and ran inside. Eddie was playing on the floor with cards. I told him, "Tell Maw I went on a walk with a friend. Be back soon!" As I ran out, I grabbed a sweater.

We took a walk down by the river at a small lake nearby. Not much was said. The lake was like glass. I could almost see my reflection in it; I did see the reflection of the trees.

We stopped, and Josef skipped a rock on the water.

"I want to learn how to do that!" I exclaimed. "Can you show me how?"

He showed me how he placed the rock in his hand and threw it. It skipped three times.

I gave it a try. My first rock plopped right into the lake. I tried a few more times without success. He then walked over and placed his hand over mine.

As he shook the back of my hand, he said, "Alice — just relax and let my hand do the work."

Well, it worked.

Together we threw a rock into the lake, and it skipped twice!

We walked side by side on a trail by the lake and talked for hours. We first started talking about the beauty of nature that surrounded us. Then, he told me that he was working at the brewery part-time, where his father worked. However, he may have to leave that job because his brother and he ran a family buggy business. It was doing quite well.

Unexpectedly, he turned to face me and asked, "Could you accompany me to a dance in a few weeks at the Weston Farmer's Hall?"

I responded, "That would be nice, but you first need to meet my father and mother."

He agreed.

Looked like it wasn't a one-way admiration. It seemed that Josef liked me — really liked me. I wondered where this would go.

The next week I would finally be graduating high school. Maw took me downtown to get my picture taken by Hugo Anton Hermann von Broich. I was honored! This was an important accomplishment for our family, for me to be the first one of the Wood children to graduate high school.

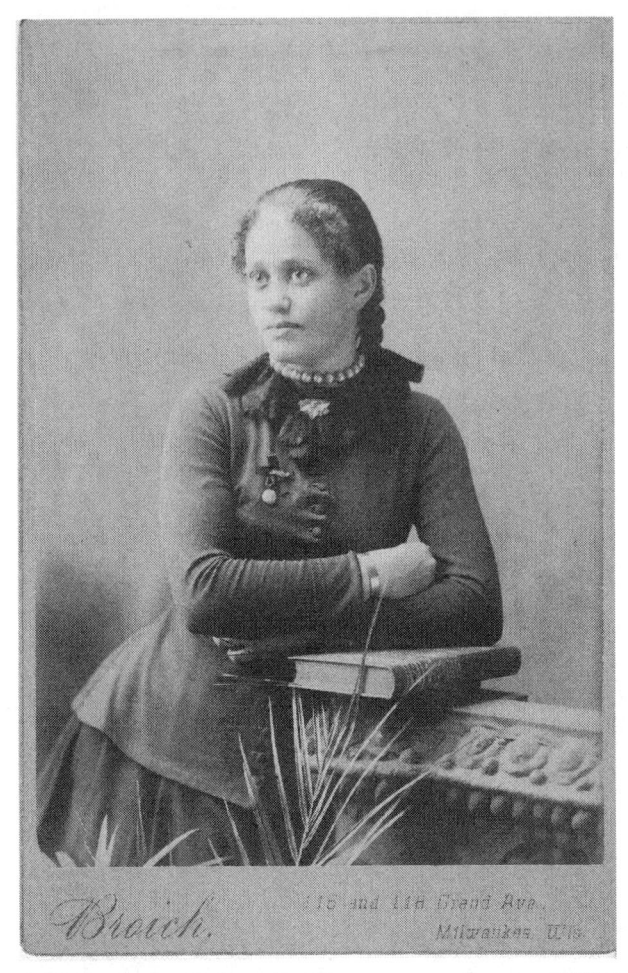

Alice Ada Wood 18 years of age 1886

Susan E. Fleming

CHAPTER 9
MOVING FORWARD:
TRICKS & SKILLS OF THE TRADE
MILWAUKEE 1886

It was official. My sister Beulah had stopped midwifing. She said never again.

So, our family decided to send her to college first at the Milwaukee State Normal School. It had been open for a couple of years. Even though they taught her primarily how to become a teacher, she would choose to do accounting once she graduated.

After graduating from high school, I found myself attending so many births. Yet, I felt like I was not being acknowledged.

Maw and Beu kept undermining my confidence. I would make one step forward and find myself falling two steps back.

I realized that they might not be aware of how I felt. I decided to confront my family.

One evening I came home, and the whole family was relaxing in our gathering room.

I decided to speak my piece.

I thundered, "Okay, family. I need to speak with you! Especially Maw and Beu."

Grandma placed her knitting down to listen and said, "Oh, this is gonna be good."

Pa murmured, "Come on, Eddie — let's go to the barn and break up the hay."

"What are you talking about, Pa?" Eddie asked. "We just did that last night?"

Pa grabbed Eddie. "Let's get out of here now!"

I immediately jumped in. "Slow down there, Pa.

You need to hear this too!"

At that point, I had everyone's attention.

"Listen," I said. "I am eighteen years old! I am a woman. You all treat me like a child."

Eddie said, "Not me, Al. I have your back." I gave Eddie a nod of acknowledgment.

"Okay," I continued. "Let me be blunt. First, I finished high school and began working full-time as a midwife. I bring money into the family pot! Yet, you continue to be hampering my confidence. I realize you have been trying to be sensitive to me since the rape. I hear ya! Maw and Beu talk away, saying Alice is too young, she can't handle that, she won't be of much help. Aren't these sayings a bit old? What is this about? Since the rape, *you* have all regressed. I did for a bit, but I can't move forward with you acting like this. For Heaven's sake — please move forward with me."

I looked at Maw and Beu. "Maw, you tell me I need to move forward on my own time. Well, here it is. My own time."

Then I addressed Pa. "Pa, I have been telling you I want to be a hunter. I love the thought of hunting, but I am beginning to realize that I don't desire to be a hunter as to be treated like you believe in Eddie. Believe in me."

I gazed at everyone in the room and declared, "I am a midwife, a woman capable of making my own decisions. In fact, I will be going to a dance with a young man named Josef. He is Johanna's older brother. As a matter of respect, he will ask Pa and Maw for permission. I am sure you will all make him feel welcome."

"What Alice is saying is true!" Grandma said.

Beu spoke up. "Alice, you are right, of course. We just want to protect you."

"Alice," Maw said. "We — or at least I — didn't realize we were regressing. Well, maybe I am wrong. I guess we are treating you like a child again. But you are right. I will welcome your man friend."

Everyone looked at Pa. Maw gave him a nudge. "Oh yeah," he said. "I will too."

Ugh, families.

As I developed my skills in helping women birth. I realized that there was an art and a science to birthing — and I needed to learn both.

Maw and Grandma each had their own style — and I would have mine.

When I brought it up, Maw suggested I help other midwives in the area. That way, I could see more differences between working styles. I agreed that this could be helpful.

It was summer, and now that I was out of school, I had plenty of time and opportunities to help other midwives.

Most of the midwives I worked with were skilled, and many were recent immigrants from Europe. A few even were like Maw and Grandma — women who had been trained through their family lines or had assisted in hospitals during the war between the states.

I soon began to realize that it was not easy working with older experienced midwives that you felt didn't have good skills — especially if they gave bad advice.

I had done enough midwifing; I could recognize good skills.

And one midwife I helped — Maude — did not have them. It was very hard to help her. I barely lasted a week with her.

First of all, she wasn't the cleanest person in town. I only saw her wash her hands *after* the babies were born. I had to talk with her.

"Maude. My Maw and I have been attending lectures at St Mary's Hospital, and the doctors and midwives from Europe suggest we wash our hands when we first arrive in the home and any time they get soiled."

"Well, aren't you a know-it-all! Look, Alice, you can ask questions, but leave the advice-giving up to me."

"Fine, but I will wash my hands," I said. The rest of the day did not go well.

She also liked the women to lie flat on their backs on tables — often dirty kitchen tables. I felt a table was more convenient for her, not the mother.

At the end of the day, while helping Maude during the actual birth, I placed gentle pressure below the mother's pelvis on the baby's head — only to have her slap my hand away. She raved that with her hands-off technique, she didn't have many tears to deal with.[16]

That was a lie. Many of her mothers did tear during birth. The tears were mostly on top where they urinated. This was quite painful for the moms.

During pushing, Maude told her ladies to hold their breaths as she counted to ten, then to bear down and push. One of the ladies who followed her instructions broke every blood vessel in her eyes. Even worse, her baby was bluer for much longer than I had seen with other births.

My worst and last day with her was when she had a lady push too soon. The woman swelled so badly that she could not push the baby out. We had to bring her to a hospital. I heard they had to do a c-section to save the mama's life. Sadly, the baby died.

Needless to say, that was the last time I helped Maude.

It wasn't all bad, though, for me. I did learn what happens when you practice poorly and what not to do.

I worked with other midwives that summer, who were more skilled and helped me improve even more. For the most part, it was an exciting time of my life.

I wanted to move out, as I was 18 years old and had finished schooling.

Maw asserted that I needed to earn money as a midwife, as you can't always depend on a man. Grandma and Maw said that I should focus on becoming a nurse, as the nursing school would open soon.

Honestly, they were more excited about schooling to become a nurse than I was. Ever since I heard there would be no maternal classes there, my interest had declined. I preferred working in the homes.
In the meantime, though, Josef would finally be coming to ask my parents if he could escort me to the dance.

A week before the dance, Josef came to meet my parents.

We gathered in the parlor. He respectfully asked them, "Mr. and Mrs. Wood, may I have the honor of taking Alice to the dance with me?"

Maw quickly responded, "Oh, Josef, we would love that."

Pa wasn't as enthusiastic. "So, Josef, tell me about your horse and buggy skills. I assume that is how you will be traveling to the dance?"

"Yes, sir," Josef said. "My father is the Lead Brewmeister at the Herman Reutelschöfer Brewery in Milwaukee. However, he has had my older brother and I managing our family horse and buggy business for several years now. He thought it would be good training for young men to run their own business."

Maw stood. "Come on, Alice, let's let the men talk." I followed her into the kitchen to help with dinner.

I saw Josef following Pa to the barn.

Oh no! What is Pa up to, for Heaven's sake?

Soon we hear the rifles shooting.

Of course — Pa was testing his shooting skills.

I spoke. "Maw, I am so embarrassed! Testing his shooting skills? Is that necessary? He lets Josef shoot at targets but will not let me. Not fair. He's always complaining about wasting ammunition."

"Alice, shooting is important for your father."

Josef and Pa both returned for dinner, laughing as they walked in.

I was glad to see Josef must have been a good shot. Or, maybe better, that Pa liked him.

A week later, Josef returned with his buggy. I gladly accompanied him to the dance. My parents decided that I didn't need a chaperone.

Perhaps, they don't know me very well, I teasingly thought, dancing the night away with Josef.

The dance was delightful.

After that, Josef and I tried to meet at least once a week.

One day, we decided to take a walk. We returned to the woods where our first date was, down by the lake.

This day was very special, as I felt we were getting closer. I made lunch and brought a blanket for our adventure. As we approached the lake, I could see it was beautiful. The rolling hills and trees were reflecting on the lake. A light breeze blew by.

We both sat down on the blanket. Soon, we relaxed and laid down together. I began to pick the grass. I think my nervousness was setting in.

Josef said, "Alice, I really do like you. You take my breath away."

I responded, "Oh Josef, I like you too. I smile more these days than ever."
Josef leaned over, and we kissed.

This was the first time I ever kissed a man I had deep feelings for. I felt a surge of energy overtaking me. *What was this?* It scared me a bit.

Josef was slightly blushing as we pulled apart. Perhaps, it was uncomfortable for him too.

Unexpectedly, I start reminiscing about the rape. I hadn't given it much thought since I had been dating Josef. When I was with him, I had better things to think about.

My logical mind stepped in.

I best tell him now, I figured.

"Josef," I said. "Wait a minute. You say you like me, but do you really know me?"

He quickly answered.

"All I know is that I feel very comfortable with you; in fact, I want to spend even more time with you, Alice."

I picked at the grass. It was hard to look at him. I needed to ask him.

"Would you like me if you knew I had a past? Would you want to spend time with a woman who was violated?"

He responded, "Alice, I would — but it sounds like you are troubled. Do you want to share something with me?"

We spent the next couple of hours lying on our backs on the blanket we had laid on the grass and talking about the violent rape I had experienced.

Josef told me that he wished he could have been there to protect me. I told him that no one can always be with me except God. I also needed to learn how to protect myself.

He told me that his mother was also raped back in Germany, by a drunken man. It was right after she was married to his father. They never found the man. His mother was taking medicine to her own mother late at night when it happened. So unexpected, just like my experience. He told me that maybe I could talk to her about this one day. I agreed.

We decided to eat lunch, but to my surprise, neither of us were hungry. We finished our date with laughing and chasing each other through the fields. It was lovely.

CHAPTER 10
BIRTHING SCIENCE:
HEADACHES & VISUAL DISTURBANCES
MILWAUKEE - 1889

Three years later, I was sent to visit Emma — the same Emma I thought was returning to Boston.

She didn't make it back. However, she did leave her husband and moved to the other side of town.

Her ex-husband headed out west; she never heard from him again.

Like many pioneer women left with children alone, she soon met and married a man willing to care for her and her two little girls. He was a Jewish man named Uri, who had a hat store in town. [B-8]   I was so happy to meet him, as he was so kind. I noticed that he had fun playing with her girls. The girls were now almost 4 and 6 years old.

They had a wooden sign hanging in the house that said *B'Sha'ah Tovah*. I was unfamiliar with this saying. I inquired, "Uri — tell me about that sign. What does it mean?"

Uri replied, "It means *at the right time* — otherwise known as *at a good hour*. In this case, it may all go well with the pregnancy."

I responded, "Very nice. Don't we all want this?"

I asked Emma, "Why are you having me come to visit you so early?" Once more, she had a midwife visit when she was only six months pregnant.

She responded, "I am getting a sharp pain in my chest, and my feet look swollen. Just like before, the baby isn't moving much."

"You might consider chewing chalk — chalk as you see in schools. If it works, you most likely have a stomach ailment."[B-17.]

I listened to her baby's heart, which was regular and fast.

I shared, "The baby's heart sounds are good. Your uterus is soft, with no contractions or bruising noted. Are you cramping or having discharge?"

"Oh, that's good," she said. "And no, no cramping or any discharge."

I asked her, "Do your hands seem swollen? They seem swollen to me."

She replied, "No, I don't reckon. Well, maybe, my rings are getting a bit tight. I have headaches but have been troubled by these for years. Nothing new to report."

I reassured her that her pregnancy was fine. Both parents were filled with joy to hear this great news.

I told her to call me back if the swelling worsened or if she had more questions. I left feeling so happy for her, her children, and her new husband. She and her children deserve to be happy and loved. God had given her a second chance at happiness.

I continued to provide midwifing to the families in town seeking care. I found this to be so rewarding most of the time.

Yet, there was plenty of sorrow.

It was interesting to see the effect moving out west with no family had on people. Often, there was no accountability; no one could call them out on their misdeeds or poor choices.

There was a reason they were calling this the *Wild West* — it was because it was. There was no law and order. Disorderly conduct prevailed. As communities formed out west, you would see that they often placed the courthouse in the center of town. This was where they used to place churches. Sheriffs would come and go as the wind blew.

Milwaukee was recognizing that evil. Soon, politicians gave the public hope by promising to bring law and order. Pa said that underneath most of the politicians' concern lay power-hungry men

motivated by fame and greed. They would dismiss the safety of the people for their personal gain.
We heard a knock one late evening when we were all in our beds.

This wasn't surprising. Our birthing business kept Maw and me quite busy.

I assured my mother, who was making to get up — "Maw, I can take care of this one. You get some sleep. You've had a rough couple of nights with birthing. You look like you'll pass out."

I open the front door to Uri. His horse was tied loosely behind him. "Hurry, Alice," he pled. "Can you come with me? Emma is in trouble."

I knew immediately that this would not end well. I told him, "I'll follow you on my horse." I quickly told Maw, "I am leaving; it's Emma. We might call in a doctor." I knew Maw needed to sit this birth out and get sleep.

Maw said, "Oh no — this birth is too early. Be safe."

I gathered my supplies and ran out to the barn to get on my horse to join him.

We took our horses down to the trail by the river. The moon lit our silent way. Not a word was spoken.

As we entered the home, I noticed a candle burning in a glass jar on a wooden table.

The warmth from the stove was dwindling as the wood fire burned down to glowing embers. The children were quiet as they lay sound asleep in their beds above, up in the loft.

Emma was propped on the couch with pillows under her arms, which seemed to ease her breathing. Immediately, as I approached her, I noticed that her swelling had increased, especially in her face.[B-18]

Her moans were broken and faint — not the sounds of a woman getting ready to birth. Next to the couch was a wooden cradle, hand-made by Uri and filled with yarn and needles. Nearby, a nearly finished knitted baby blanket had been thrown on the floor.

Uri recounted what was happening.

"Emma had recently been bothered by the stomach flu, as she had sharp pains in her belly and was beginning to vomit. Her unbearable headaches had become more persistent, and she began to see flickering lights. She reassured me that these ailments would pass. They haven't. I made sure to keep a vial of opium nearby."[B-19]

I attempted to speak with Emma, but her weakened state was evident. She answered with a simple nod or a squeeze of my hand. Her breathing was labored. I could hear crackling sounds coming from her chest as she breathed. I knew her lungs were filling with fluid.

I lifted the blanket and saw a pool of dark blood dripping from her birth opening. As I examined her abdomen, I saw no bruises. But her belly felt a bit rigid, not like a normal pregnancy. [B-13] Her pain seemed more severe on the upper side of her belly. I noticed her face and hands were swollen.

I had to figure this out.

I offered to help Uri build up the fire. I went outside to gather wood outside from the wood pile.

In the silence of the outdoors, I delved into my experiences of previous births.

What were the clues?

During her last pregnancy, she had a rigid belly and was bleeding dark red blood.[B-13] It was related to trauma from her husband kicking her. My gut said Uri would not hurt her; I didn't see any bruising.

This time seemed more serious as her breathing and pains overcame her. Why was she so swollen? Most pregnant women have swelling, mostly in their feet. This was so different. Her swelling was in her hands and face. I walked back into the house with a bag full of wood.

As I returned to the house with wood, Uri greeted me at the door. He was so desolate. Tears were in his eyes. He pled, "Please help my Emma. Please."

I was in despair. What could I do? I answered, "I will try my best…Uri, we need to call in a doctor."

Together, we walked over to Emma. Her body was failing. But just then, things started moving quickly.

I looked under the blanket and saw a baby's head protruding.

I bent over to help remove the baby.

I softly announced, "It is a boy."

His skin was completely white, except for his mouth, which was dark purple since blood had pooled there. His tender skin was peeling off his back. There was no life in this baby. I decided to cut the white floppy cord right away. No need to wait. I cleaned him up with the few rags from my bag. [B-20]

The warm baby quickly became cool to the touch.

I gently wrapped him in the new baby blanket Emma had just knitted. Then I handed the sweet baby to the grief-stricken new father.

Uri tenderly proclaimed, "He shall be called 'Elijah', like my father, which means *Jehovah is my God*."

He walked over to the rocking chair while holding his baby — his son. He sat and rocked back and forth, mourning his loss.

I stayed with Emma, waiting for the placenta to expel. I could hear her weakly gasping. As her placenta expelled, she started to have fits.[B-21]

Soon after, every orifice in Emma's dying body started to drain blood. The gate was open. Every hair follicle began to be marked with blood. Blood dripped out of her eyes and mouth. [B-22]

Uri laid his son in the cradle he had made and walked over to comfort Emma as her dying body became less responsive. Her lungs rattled with congestion as her breathing decreased.

Then, in a moment, she stopped taking breaths.

Emma had died.

Uri carried her lifeless body to the rocking chair as he wept.

I walked over and reloaded the stove. I asked Uri if he would like me to clean the couch to have a place to lay Emma. He agreed that it would be nice. After I finished cleaning, he laid Emma down on the couch. He told me he needed to go outside and walk. I told him to take his time, and that I would help clean and dress Emma. He laid a clean outfit for Emma to wear before he left.

I finished cleaning Elijah and dressed him in the fresh outfit Emma had made for him. I gently laid him back in the cradle, then started tending to Emma. I looked at the dress for Emma that Uri had left and decided the only way I could get it on her was to cut the back, tuck it around her, then pin it together.

Uri returned. "Alice, can you stay in the house, as the children will wake soon? I just talked to the local undertaker, who is also my rabbi. He agreed to receive Emma and their baby during this early morning hour."

I told him that, of course, I would.

I helped Uri as he carried his lovely Emma to the buggy outside. I walked out to the buggy and laid Elijah in her arms. I couldn't help but to tuck a warm blanket around both of them. I waved goodbye as I walked back to the house. My eyes were filled with tears.

My heart sank as I felt such sorrow for the family. After I finished cleaning the house, I lay down by the fire to get some sleep.

Soon, I saw the light piercing through the curtains. The morning was here. I opened my eyes, and two little girls were looking right at me.

They had climbed down from the loft by themselves. The youngest started crying. "Mommy. I want my mommy." The oldest daughter comforted her little sister.

I stood up and made them breakfast. They were hungry. I did not mention their mommy.

Soon, Uri returned. The little girls cried out as they ran over to his arms, "Daddy, Daddy!"

He brought the girls to the couch and talked with them. Soon, they were all crying. I couldn't hear what he said. He was hugging them gently as I walked out the door. I felt the girls didn't know exactly what had happened, but they felt Uri's sorrow and cried with him.

I mounted my horse and headed home. I anguished as I contemplated what life would become for those little girls and Uri.

I bitterly regretted telling Uri and Emma just a few

weeks ago that her pregnancy was fine. Could I have done anything better to prevent such a tragic outcome? I soon arrived home.

I walked into the house with tears in my eyes. Grandma and Maw greeted me as I entered the house. They knew what had happened without me saying a word. They both hugged me.

Maw said, "Alice, you get some rest. We can talk later."

I walked up to the loft and laid my head down.

Several hours later, I awakened still in a daze. I walked into the kitchen and wept.

I told Maw and Grandma exactly what happened. "I feel so hopeless. There was nothing I could do. What will happen to the little girls?"

They acknowledged my deep sorrow.

I explained that I had just gone to their home a couple of weeks earlier, and all was well, except for Emma's swelling hands and persistent headache. I explained that Emma shared that the headaches were common, and she hardly recognized the swelling, even though I had. They both shared with me their experiences of similar cases.

Grandma says one of the doctors she met at a lecture in Milwaukee called this *eclampsia*, the most serious type of convulsive disorder developing during pregnancy. It was often related to kidney disease.

Grandma shared, "Alice, there is not much you can do for these pregnant ladies with fits. If you have chloroform, sprinkle it on a handkerchief and hold it to the mother's nose. And make sure to call a doctor if there is time. If the child survives this tormenting labor, keep the baby away from the mother. The mother may injure the baby as she has fits."

I appreciated them telling me how to apply good skills, but this did not help my deep-felt sorrow and, more so, my guilt. They both confirmed that, most likely, there was nothing I could have done.

Several months go by, and I saw the little girls are still with Uri as I watched them riding in his buggy. I also noticed he has a new woman friend. Perhaps, they will marry.

I eventually heard that Uri's rabbi and his wife had been so helpful, as they always found care for the children as Uri managed his hat store in town. I was amazed by his commitment to the little girls. I had thought that for sure he wouldn't take care of them. I imagine all three would share the grief of losing Emma for many years.

CHAPTER 11
HEALING:
CAN A HUNT BRING ME PEACE?
1890

I lay in my bed and pondered.

I realized it had been a year since Emma had passed, yet I still would find myself distraught over her.

It started to affect me.

I would also like to say I had gotten over the rape. I never did. That tormenting experience had left me more vulnerable than ever.

After Emma's death, I had begun to lose confidence in myself. I felt so out of control. Initially I felt numb. I even felt myself denying the experience. Grandma and Maw were so helpful as they were always there to listen.

I longed to be with Josef, but he had recently travelled to Chicago with his father to pick up a few more horses and buggies. They would be talking with other men about expanding their business. It could be several months before I saw him again.

I got ready and went down the ladder. I met Maw and Grandma for breakfast.

Grandma said, "Alice you look distraught. Are you missing your Josef?"

"Oh, that is part of what is going on."

"Well, tell us, girl. How are you feeling?"

"I wish I was stronger, like you two ladies. You are both so tough. I must admit that the death of Emma and the rape still linger in my thoughts. I can't seem to shake them."

Maw so wisely told me, "Alice, I need to be honest with you. Know that often, victims don't heal. As you have seen, most people in this world are suffering. Like I have said before, you need to move forward. You are focused on what has happened. You need to direct your focus on solutions. You will need to deal with these devastating trials in your life on your own, and in your own time."

I listened to her.

Grandma said, "*Put on the Armor of God that you may resist the schemes of the devil.* It says it right here in our Bible. I know you can do it, Alice."

"I will do this. For you, Grandma, I will put on the armor of God. Like you said Maw, I will direct my focus on solutions, on my own time."

November came.

I decided to move forward by talking with Pa.

I planned to tell him of my dreams and my fears -— how I had longed to be a hunter.

One night, I pled with him. "Pa, please take me out for a hunt with you. More importantly, I need to get my own rifle and then learn how to shoot it."

Pa seemed confused. "Alice, everyone in this house knows how to shoot a rifle."

I responded, "I am talking about shooting a gun with precision."

Pa confronted me with the truth, "Alice, does this have to do with your horrid experience you suffered last June?"

I answered, "Kind of. But you know I have always wanted to go hunting with you."

Pa declared, "Alice, yes, I know, but having your own rifle? Did you hear about the young girl who was walking with her rifle for protection? A transient man grabbed it from her and shot her dead. There are plenty of dangerous travelers looking to steal from others as they head west."

I replied, "Okay, maybe not my own rifle. But I do want to learn how to shoot. Shoot like I said, with precision."

Pa settled with me. "Okay, I can teach you. But I am not going to waste my ammunition on some crazy targets. Let's go next Saturday to the wetlands. I have a few days. I hear there are still deer out there."

I was so happy. Finally, Pa would take me hunting. I have longed for this day to come.

Early one morning several days later, just Pa and I rode our horses into the edge of the forest. We brought a pack horse with us. We tied the horses up and set up camp. That night, we sat around a fire as Pa prepared me for the hunt.

"Alice," he said. "Tomorrow we will leave camp and walk into the forest. Our goal is to locate where the bucks are. I always go for the bucks or old does, since we want the young deer to reproduce. It is truly the circle of life. How are you feeling about shooting and killing a deer?"

I calmly retorted, "I am ok. I haven't given it much thought."

Pa laughed. "Well, you better give it much thought. You are taking away a life, the life of that deer. Always ask yourself, is it rightful to kill? Do we need food, or is there danger?"

I pondered what he said. We spend the next hour discussing the circle of life. Our lives depend on food and deer are part of our food source. Deer provides food for our existence. I finally proclaimed, "I need to be thankful for taking the deer's life."

Pa answered, "Yes, you do. A few hunters I know say a prayer to thank *Heavenly Father* for giving us the deer's life.[B-28] Does this appeal to you?"

I nodded.

He continued. "We honor the animal and realize they lost their life to feed our families. We are essentially the top predator in the food chain and the deer view us the same as a wolf bear or mountain lion. Do they give themselves to one of them? They just want to keep surviving. Often times when I harvest an animal, I think this animal had no clue this would be their last day of life and it truly saddens me. I attribute that loss to a blessing from God who provided the animal for me. Interestingly, on days I don't harvest, I still thank God for allowing me to be in the beautiful world he created and return home safely to my family." B-28

"That was beautiful Pa. Truly a meaningful pursuit."

"Well then, it sounds like you are getting closer to be ready. We can talk more in the morning."

Early the next morning, we proceeded to tread into the dark woodlands. I felt the falling leaves crunch under my feet as I trudged through the thinning forest. I felt the chill in the air that lingered from the blackened nights. I saw the frost on the ground as it rose as a fine mist.

Soon, the sun warmed the ground. As I stepped through, I saw rotting fruit that had fallen to the ground, only to be bruised by the hardened earth, and soon to be forgotten as it decayed into the soil. A somber reminder of death, which will come to us all.

Yet, there was a foretaste that new life was on the horizon, as it was deer rutting season. The rut-crazed bucks get little sleep as they searched for the scent of a doe in heat. Following those deer were the hunters. I was now one of those hunters.

Pa was a seasoned hunter, and I was eager to learn. I would learn the art of hunting, but mostly the challenge and pursuit of the hunt.

Motivated bucks break through the forest leaving broken trees as a trail for hunters to follow. We tallied our hits alongside our misses each day. We waited to ambush our prize as the bucks ran through the river grasses of the nearby woods.

One time, while we were waiting, a doe ran before us. Papa whispered, "See that doe running through the forest? Do you notice the sound she is making? A buck is sure to follow and lock on to her. Let's go over to that hill over there. There is a marsh on the edge of the forest. There in the marsh, we will wait for the buck to rest after he tends to the doe."

We quietly hiked over to the marsh, by a big tree. Pa glared at me when I tried to speak. I realized that we needed to be silent.

Two hours later, just like Pa said, a large buck strolled into the marsh snorting and blowing out air as he found a resting place. Unbeknownst to the buck, it was his death march.

With Pa's guidance, I aimed and made the shot.

Right into the buck's shoulder.

The startled buck took off, only to collapse soon after.

Pa was astonished, "Well Alice, it looks like you are a natural. You have a good eye; such precision."
I did it.

We shot and killed two more. It was a good hunt.

We gutted the deer.

Pa said, "Look at you, girl, digging right in. Cutting and degutting. You got it! Let's go bring in our pack horse."

I was thrilled.

Pa and I had a wonderful time. Under his guidance, I was able to shoot deer for our winter stors. More importantly, I learned how to shoot with precision. The hunting expedition ended on the river's bluff in the west.

We returned home sporting our hunting gear, which we had worn for days, and carrying in our prized deer to add to our collection, to cure and provide meat for our family to last through the cold and desolate winter.

Anticipating our return, Beu and Eddie prepared the barn for our return by filling the hay boxes and water troughs for our horses. They had heard the faint neighs of our horses as a signal that we were nearby.

We unloaded the three deer off the pack horses into the cool back room of the barn to protect the kill from ravenous predators. Pa threw a rope over the large beams to hang the deer. As we tended to the hanging deer, we pulled a few tenderloins for our evening supper.

Several days later, we would return to process the deer by salting the meat.

Maw celebrated our hunt with gracious thanks, adding the fresh venison tenderloins to the stew pot. The whole family expressed gratitude as we blessed our meal that night.

The hunt with Pa was healing.

I realized my desire to hunt, also had to do with having control of my life.

With hunting, I am in control. I do not have to succumb to fate, like I do with midwifing. I decide when and which deer will die. With midwifing, I am often lost for options. Bringing life into this world was not as simple as I thought it would be.

I anguished when I thought of Emma, a woman whose life was cut short. She was robbed of so many opportunities — most of all, never being able to see her own daughters grow. Finally, she had a man who was by her side and loved her girls as much as she did — and her body mysteriously took her life away.

I was torn. Would I be a better hunter than a midwife? I could help feed the people of my community.

I needed time to decide my fate.

Within time, I decided to go back to midwifing.

I looked at midwifing with a new perspective. I didn't always have answers. But from what I had seen, neither did other midwives. Even doctors didn't always know what was happening.

I pledged to give my best and to be by mothers' sides as they birth. It really felt good to know I could serve others in a meaningful way. It helped me to rid my self-pity. Like Maw had said so many times before, there were many people suffering — a lot more than I could ever imagine.

Our family also started going to church more routinely. It was good to belong to a group of people trying to make lives better for women. We could all be there to help each other. As a midwife, I often found myself assisting women with their relationships as well as birth.

Susan E. Fleming

CHAPTER 12
CREATING LARGE BABIES:
LOOKING LIKE A TURTLE
MILWAUKEE - 1890

I would like to say that there was no more sorrow. But there was. There would always be, with more to come.

Yet throughout the sorrow, I witnessed slivers of happiness and great joy.

One day, I was called upon to help two sisters. They worked at the German bakery in town known as *Becker's Bäckerei*. Their father owned the bakery. Their names were quite interesting: Candi and Lolli Becker. They were both unmarried and in their mid-thirties. They shared an apartment above the bakery. To their surprise, they were both pregnant.

This was an outrage for their father Herr Martin Becker and his wife Hedwig. They were livid. The girls claimed they were just as shocked. They claimed that they never had relations with any man.

I went up to their flat and knocked. Candi answered the door. She was the oldest, I had been told.

"You must be Alice; Come on in. And this is my sister Lolli; her real name is Lollipop."

I smile. But I couldn't believe my ears. *Who in their right mind would have a girl named Lollipop?*

I notice candy dishes on every table.

Not surprising, I must admit I thought.

I settled in and evaluated them.

They were both very large. To look at them, I would not even think they were pregnant, just overweight. I tried to get a bit of a history.

Their stories were quite hard to follow as they answered for each other.

"So, Candi and Lolli" I finally asked. "Who would you like me to check first?"

Immediately, they pointed at each other and said in unison, "Her!"

They giggled like grammar-school girls.

At that moment, I recognized this was not going to be easy. I needed to take charge with these silly ladies.

I pulled out my in-charge midwife voice, "Candi, you'll go first. Lie here on the couch — and Lolli, you stay seated at the table. I can only talk with you one at a time; do you understand?"

"I do!" they said, again in unison.

Seriously?

Candi lay on the couch. I pulled up a chair and sat beside her. "Candi, when was your last bleed?" I asked. "Can you tell me, when did you first notice you were pregnant?"

Lolli began to answer. "It was…"

I shot her a stern gaze — the look that Maw would give us kids growing up. Lolli immediately became quiet.

Candi responded. "Well, my last bleed was a long time ago, and about 6 months ago we — I mean I — got really sick. I was vomiting every day. I thought we — sorry, I — had some type of stomach ailment. But after a couple weeks, this diminished. And just a few weeks ago, I started to feel movement in my belly. And the nausea had returned. I thought, here it goes again, my stomach ailment has returned, this time with gas. I find myself getting thirsty and using the latrine all the time. Most of all, I am extremely tired." [B-23]

"I would like to hear this from you," I said. "Do you recall having relations with a man, say, eight months ago?

"Tell her, Candi, tell her!!" called out Lolli.

"Shhh, Lolli, you speak too much. Ignore her, Alice."

"I will not be quiet anymore. We need help. The only way Alice can help us is if we tell the truth. I am tired of being so secretive," cried out Lolli.

Candi sighed. "Oh, all right. Alice, can we trust you? You must not tell our parents, especially Father. He would kill us."

"Go on," I said.

"Well, as you know, we are adult women. We have desires. Lolli and I always stay at the *Bäckerei* late to clean up. And this delivery man named Heinrich would make weekly deliveries right before we closed. He seemed to like me. So, I invited him up to our apartment. It wasn't long after that our relations started. He started making deliveries every other day. Lolli could hear us. At first, she was angry. But before I knew it, he was taking turns with both of us. This lasted for about three months. Every other day."

"He was so manly! Ooh, how I miss him and his deliveries," called out Lolli.

"Shhh!" Candi hushed her before continuing. "Then one night, a lady came into our shop while he was making his delivery of flour and sugar. She hit him in the head with a rolling pin. She was his wife. We didn't know that he was married. I have no idea of what she knew. Well, that was the last we saw of him. The next day we had a different delivery man."

"He wasn't as friendly," exclaimed Lolli.

"Okay," I said. "So, your babies will have the same father."

They both nodded their heads yes.

This was getting complicated.

I spent the next few hours evaluating them. First, they were complaining of the same things, which were nausea, thirst, and frequent urination. They both complained of being tired.[B-23] I was not sure what was causing this, but I would ask Maw and Grandma when I got home.

According to them, Candi and Lolli really didn't start gaining more weight until three months ago. I could hear a faint heartbeat with my pinard on Lolli, and I could feel the baby move with Candi.

Could it be they would be expecting soon? I believed so. I also believed their father knew they weren't telling the truth about having relations with a man.

That evening at home, I talked with Maw and Grandma about the sisters. They listened attentively and did chuckle a bit.

Maw told me, "In New York during the war, an Indian fellow told me that in his tribe if they had people being extra thirsty or peeing all the time, they would take the urine and drip it on the floor. If the next day they noticed ants drinking the urine, they knew there was sugar in it. They called it *honey urine*."[B-23]

Grandma put her two cents in. "It makes sense to me, if you're peeing all the time and the ants are eating it. Stop taking in all that sugar."

"You might be right Grandma; there were candy bowls everywhere in their rooms, and they were both overweight." I shared. "What should I do?"

Maw responded. "Not sure what you should do Alice — just be careful. I have had trouble help birthing babies from extra-large women. The babies seem to get stuck."

"I've seen that too," shared Grandma.

I wasn't excited to hear that news.

Several weeks later, a courier appeared at our door in the early morning. "It is time," he told us. "It is one of the Becker sisters."

I knew immediately I would need help. Maw had just left an hour ago for the birth of twins — and even took Beu with her.

I looked over, and there was Grandma sitting in her comfy chair.

I pointed to her. "Grandma French, you are coming with me!"

"Me?" Grandma asked.

"Is there anybody else in the house named Grandma French?" I smiled.

Slowly, Grandma got ready. I helped her with her barn clothes and help her put on an apron. I then told her, "Don't worry; we'll take the buggy."

When we arrived, I tied our horse Sadie to the post in front of the *Bäckerei*. Then, I helped Grandma step down as we grabbed our bags.

We walked into the *Bäckerei*.

Frau Becker met us at the door and welcomed us in. "Alice, Ich bin so froh, dass du hier bist. Lolli ist bereit zur Geburt und Candi ist an ihrer Seite. Nach oben gehen," she said, and pointed for us to go up the stairs. I translated for grandma, "She said, I'm so glad you're here. Lolli is ready to give birth, and Candi is by her side. Go upstairs."

As I head towards the stairs, I introduced my grandmother, "Oh wunderbar, vielen Dank, Frau Becker. Ich habe meine Großmutter Mary mitgebracht. Sie ist auch Hebamme."

Frau Becker gave us a nod of acknowledgement coupled with a welcoming smile.

As we approached the upstairs door, I could hear screaming. I tell Grandma, "It's Lolli. I imagine she is quite scared. We will need to focus on calming her down."

Inside the apartment, Lolli was lying flat on a bed, thrashing back & forth. I quickly took charge, sitting next to her on the bed.

"Lolli, this is Alice. Look at me. Let's breathe together."

Lolli cried out, "Ich kann nicht! Ich möchte das nicht tun. Hilf mir! Hilf mir jetzt." Grandma, she says she wants help and can't do this."

She was completely out of control.

I grabbed both of her hands and held them down. "Lolli, look at me. The baby is coming and will soon be here. You need to slow down your breathing."

Lolli began to relax and started speaking English. "Okay. Okay," she said. "Just take it out. Take it out now. I beg of you. I don't vant to have a baby!"

"Breathe with me. In and out. In and out. you got it. Grandma, shall we cool some washcloths for her forehead?" I asked.

"Sounds good to me, Alice. She is not relaxed enough to give birth. Let's help her sit up in bed. And put a pillow or blanket under her knees. This will prop her into a sitting position. It will help her unwind."

We spent the next hour helping Lolli relax. Grandma started massaging her feet. It seemed to help. Candi helped me stoke up the fireplace, as the room was quite cold when we got there.

Grandma taught Candi how to use counting on her fingers to help Lolli relax and breathe. When Candi held up three fingers, Lolli breathed in three times. With two fingers, two times, and so on, and so on. This trick really helped. Lolli started to focus, and it helped her control her breathing.

We prepared the couch with fresh newspapers and cheesecloth. The room was darkened except the glow of the fireplace timbers. We make sure Lolli had plenty of water to drink. We make a tea from lavender for her to sip on. As Lolli relaxed, her contractions started to increase. She desired to lay down rather than to stay sitting upright.

Eventually, she felt the urge to push. After twenty minutes of nothing happening, we decided to visually examine her to make sure she was progressing.
I grabbed the oil lamp, "Look here Grandma — the baby's head emerges and retracts. Like a turtle.[B-24] Could it be a short cord; should I get ready for a somersault?"

"I don't believe so, Alice," Grandma said. "I don't see excessive bleeding. Let's apply a cloth soaked in cold water and roll her over on her knees and elbows and see if that helps."

Lolli was reluctant to roll over, but together with Candi and Grandma and me, we repositioned her with her head down and bottom up.

We applied the cold cloth to her bottom to reduce the swelling. We soon saw the turtling dwindle, and then saw progression of the head as she pushed.

"Ok, Lolli, I can see red hair — a few more pushes and we will have a baby!"

The whole room was filled with relief and excitement.

"Ok," I told Candi and Grandma. "As I catch the baby, help Lolli roll on her back and lift her head."

The baby came out — and just as I asked, Candi and Grandma helped Lolli onto her back. I looked down at the sweet little baby girl.

I announced, "It's a girl!"

Candi and Lolli cried out in excitement. I smiled.

I noticed the baby did seem quite large and was struggling to breathe more than usual.

Lolli started to be fearful. "Why is she gurgling?"

"Don't fret," I urged her. "Let me dry her off some more, then let's place her on your chest, like we talked about a couple weeks ago."

The baby began to pink up as I dried her off. The baby belted out an enormous, big cry. A sense of pure joy filled the room.

Lolli announced, "I will call her Rachael. Like a lamb. Since she is innocent and beautiful."

I told her that Rachael was a beautiful name.

After an hour, everything was cleaned up. Candi went downstairs to get her parents.

"It's a girl," I heard Candi say. "Lolli named her Rachael. Why don't you come up to see your grandchild?"

At first, they were both reluctant. Soon, the girls' mama

Hedwig decided to come up.

"I don't know about you Martin, but I am going up," I heard her say in German. "Do as you please."

Even though Herr Becker showed reluctance, he decided to follow Hedwig upstairs.

They both glowed with joy as they lay eyes on the beautiful new baby. The baby looked so much like Lolli with her dark, amber-red hair.

Looks like Rachel has brought the family together.

As we rode home in the buggy, I gave Grandma my appreciation.

To my surprise, Grandma commended me.

"Alice, you have arrived," she said. "You are a compassionate and caring midwife. You are very smart as you make decisions. My mother and sisters would be proud of you. Look how you were able to calm down that anxious woman birthing."

I was full of joy, as my family is not very generous with compliments.

I replied, "Oh Grandma, I couldn't have done it without you. Your recommendation to turn her over was perfect. You knew exactly what to do."

"Not exactly," Grandma admitted.

"What do you mean?"

"Turning over on all fours is just my go-to when all else fails."

We both chuckled as we rode home.

"Alice, did you figure what was holding you back from becoming a midwife?"

"Yes, I did. You were right, it was not my age."

"So, what was it then?"

"When I went hunting with Pa, I had a real eye-opener. I realized that — unlike with hunting — with birthing, 'skill alone' will not result in good outcomes. With hunting, you are in charge of which deer dies and which one lives. Whereas, with birthing, only the good Lord in Heaven is in charge. I have had to learn on developing my faith. Knowing, if I give my best, that I shall not have to fear."

I looked at her. "It was my hatred of giving up control, that would have gotten me. It is still hard — especially when there is tragedy like with Emma, or my first birth. But I am getting better every day."

She smiled and nodded. "Nice to hear, Alice."

"Yes, I have grown to love my calling of being a midwife."

Several weeks later, we came back to help Candi birth her baby.

She had a little boy, whom she named Martin, after her father.

Again, it was a hard birth when it came to pushing. We turned her on all fours to facilitate the birth. We did not notice any turtling.

Susan E. Fleming

Alice Ada Wood: Midwife Apprentice

CHAPTER 13
STANDING WITH MY LOVE:
CAN HE PROTECT ME?
MILWAUKEE – 1891

I had longed to be with my Josef. He had been gone for several months.

I was overjoyed when he returned.

We decided to spend nearly every day together over the next few weeks. It was lovely.

One day, Josef and I traveled into nearby Westown, as he needed to pick up some new wheels for their horse buggies.

This part of town was filled with German breweries. They called this place the German Athens of America.

We parked in front of the Carriage supply store. Josef told me, "Alice, stay here. I will only be a minute."

Well, half an hour later, he still had not returned. I began to worry. Most of the stores on the street were closing.

I got out of the buggy, as I needed to walk a bit.

An intoxicated man waddled on over and slurred some words at me. "Oh, pretty lady, you've been out here quite a long time without your man friend. Perhaps he has found better fish in the sea."

I tried my best to ignore him — but he grabbed my arm. My heart sank.

Not again.

I immediately pulled my arm away. I looked him in the eyes and demanded, "Stop it right now!"

At the same time Josef stepped out of the store. I could see the anger in Josef's eyes. He stomped over to the drunken man and confronted him.

"You heard the lady; she said stop it," he growled.

The stranger man yelled, "She's no lady; she just an unwanted dollymop."

I couldn't help but think that *dollymop* was a strange name for a whore; why would anyone use that useless name?

Useless or not, the word seemed to cause Josef's blood to boil. I placed my hand on Josef's shoulder. "His words mean nothing to me," I said. "Let's walk away."

Well, Josef did not listen. The fight began.

The people on the street stopped to watch the fight. Josef's strength was evident. He threw the stranger on the ground. He tramped on over and grabbed the stranger man by the neck and threw his body into the horse trough.

After it had settled, Josef took my arm and steered me to our buggy.

Then, the unthinkable happened.

The drunken man shot Josef in the back. The bullet knocked Josef to the ground.

The man started laughing. "So, you thought your man could save you, pretty one. Not no more."

I knelt by Josef, too shocked to cry out. During the fall he hit his head on the buggy's metal seat. He was unconscious, his head gushing blood.

I looked up and the stranger was walking towards us, recklessly waving his gun around.

Will he now shoot me? I surely don't trust him.

I glanced over. I saw Josef's pistol.

Should I?

What was the alternative?

I reached into Josef's holster and grabbed his pistol.

My heart was racing; my hands were shaking. The crowds of people are staring.

I thought of the hunt. I asked myself, is it rightful to kill?

Is there danger?

Without a doubt. The decision was made.

Aim for the lung.

I stood up with both hands on the gun, pointing it at the intoxicated man. As the drunken man stumbled towards me, he tried to persuade me to put the gun down. "Put it down, sweet thing. You hear me." But as he spoke, he raised his own gun.

I said a quick prayer. Then addressed the man: "I hear you," I sneered. "I don't need a man to save me. I will do that myself."

I shot him. With precision. In the left shoulder. Through his ribs. Into his lungs.

He collapsed.

A man from the crowd ran over to check on the fallen stranger man. He announced, "He's dead."

 There was silence among the crowd.

A woman pointed to me. "She killed him."

I looked around in despair.

The crowd was silent. What happens next?

To my surprise, the crowed started clapping!

They yelled, "Good shot, pretty lady."

Well, that should be fine, then.

I turned to Josef. His face was pale as he regained consciousness.

My mind started racing. I remembered Grandma's saying: *If the face is pale raise the tail. If the face is red, raise the head.*

I grabbed a blanket from the back of the buggy, and raised his legs. A lady from the crowd gave me her shawl to wrap around his head to help stop the bleed.

Meanwhile, several men had gone to get the Sheriff.

The Sheriff walked over. "Several witnesses have told me the story. We have a consensus. You are not guilty. This was clearly a case of self-defense. Be on your way."

The people in the crowd started clapping! Then, they raced over to help me. I was given one blanket for Josef to lie on, and another one to keep his shivering body warm. Some people helped me to bandage him.

The bleeding stopped. He seemed to be feeling slightly better.

The men from the crowd offer to help me lift Josef into the back of his buggy.

Josef scoffed at the idea of getting help into the buggy. He stated, "I can make it myself."

He stepped up to the buggy and sat next to me.

I wouldn't let him drive, at least. I was taking us straight home. Maw and Grandma would help me treat him.

As I approached our home, I saw Eddie outside.

I yelled, "Eddie we need help fast! Go get Maw & Pa."

Eddie saw Josef all bandaged up. He ran inside and brought the folks outside. Together we walked with Josef into the house and laid him on our couch.

I gave them the bare bones of the story, and promised to give more once we made sure he was all right.

Maw and Grandma examined him.

Maw stated, "The bullet did enter, and is in the right side of his back. I can see it's lodged in between the ribs. I think most of the bleeding and his unconsciousness came from his head injury. He will have quite a knot there. I recommend some cool cloths to his head tonight. Keep his head elevated. You can stay the night, Josef. Pa and Eddie will ride out and notify your parents before the town does. My gut says leave the bullet alone. What do you think, Grandma?"

Grandma was decisive, "Absolutely *leave it alone*. I have seen much more damage as people try to extract the bullets. The heat of the bullet seems to stop bleeding and diseases of the flesh. Just keep your dirty hands away from there and keep it clean and covered. Check on it daily. During the war I had a few men who had walked into the hospital in New York with days old healing gunshot wounds, that no one had touched. They looked quite clean. I told them to leave and head home. Hospitals were quite dirty."

Pa agreed with the decision.

I proceeded to tell them the whole story. It was when I got to the part of shooting the man, that I looked at Pa with tears in my eyes.

"I looked at Josef's gun and decided to grab it and shoot the stranger. As I aimed, I thought of deer hunting. I asked myself, was this shot necessary? And I decided it was."

Pa spoke out. "I'm sure it was. Well done, Alice. Most likely, you hit his heart too. Being that he fell to his death so fast. This side of town is becoming wilder every day we are here."

"I don't feel like it was well done. Even though the Sheriff said I wasn't in trouble because it was clearly self-defense. I took away a life."

"That life could have been yours. You made the right move; you are heroic," said Pa.

I still felt a bit ashamed. Not heroic.

Later that evening, Josef told me how grateful he was for my quick actions. My family had told him the whole story. We could both have been killed, he said. He went on to say how incredible I was.

I thought to myself, I didn't feel incredible. I told him, "Actually, I feel despondent taking away a life of another. Even in those dire circumstances."

Josef looked sad... And much of the guilt seemed to dissolve when Josef smiled at me.

I had saved him.

Still, we decided to be more cautious when we traveled in the industrial side of town.

It was becoming quite unruly.

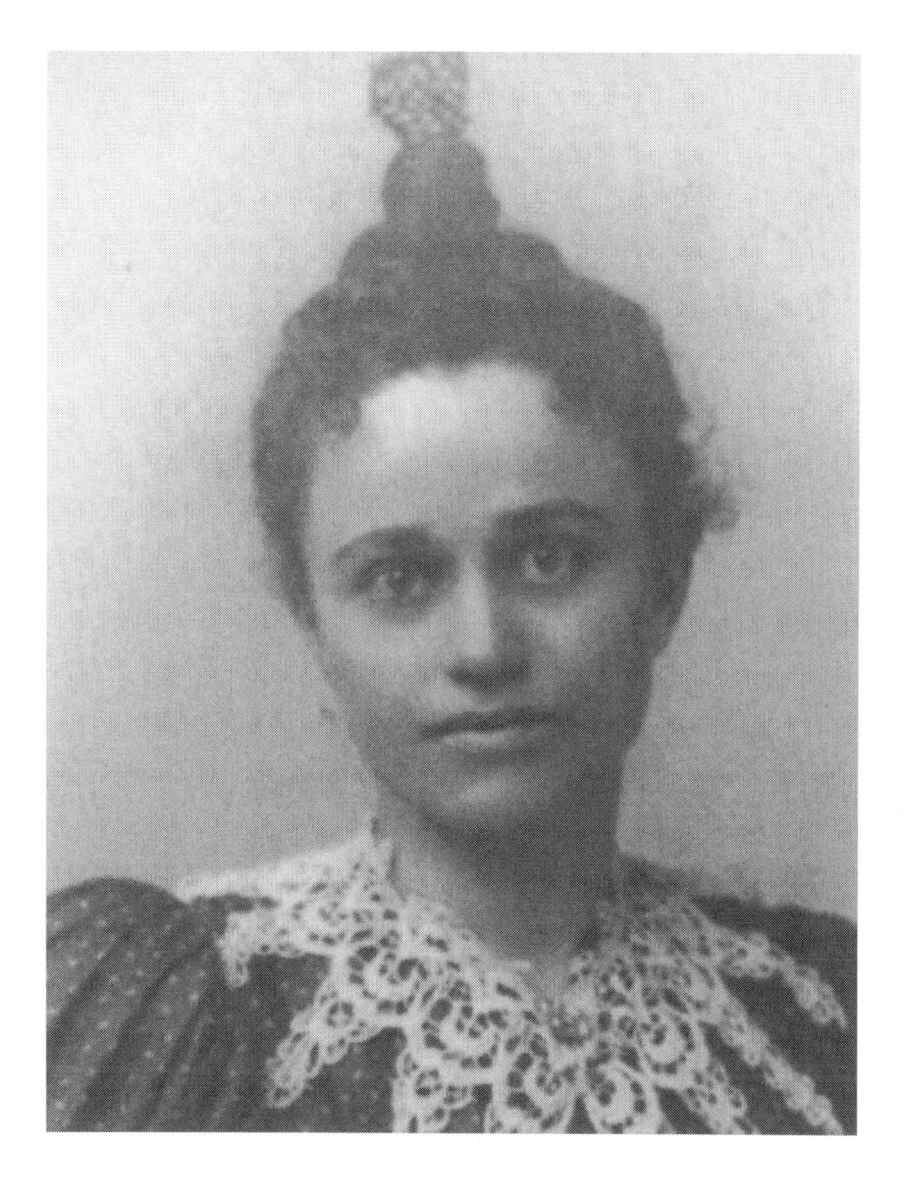

Alice in her mid 20s. Early to Mid 1890s
Milwaukee Wisconsin.

Alice Ada Wood: Midwife Apprentice

CHAPTER 14
FINDING PEACE:
COMING FULL CIRCLE
MILWAUKEE – 1892

It was a peaceful evening at home. Grandma had gone out with Beu to visit her new school and to watch a play in town called *A Doll's House*. Meanwhile, Pa and Eddie were meeting with a hunting group for young men. Unfortunately, Josef had to cancel his dinner plans with us due to an ill horse. So, it was just Maw and me at home.

Maw looked at me with a smirk. "Not much happening. It's a quiet night."

I looked at her with shame. "Maw, what the heck are you saying, woman?"

We both had a good laugh!

It was inevitable, soon we heard a knock on the door. I opened the door and there stood Albert. "Good evening, ladies. Long time, no see. There is a woman in need of help with a birth at Gertie's place. May I have the privilege of taking you lovely ladies there tonight in my charming new carriage?"

Maw and I looked at each other with a smile. Maw said, "Sure, why not? It has been a long time. Alice, may I assist you with birthing tonight?"

"I would love to have you as my assistant. Albert, we will be ready in minutes."

"I will wait in the buggy for both of you."

I checked out the birthing bag and grabbed a few medications, just in case. We were ready in no time.

We stepped up on the buggy, and away we went. Maw and I had a great discussion how to handle our upcoming situation. We knew that we wouldn't know much until we got there.

Albert helped us step down off the buggy. As usual, he agreed to wait down the alley at Marty's Inn, for a drink. He reminded us to send him a message if it would take a long time. If it would, he could come back later.

We walked down the alley, and it looked very quiet. Very strange for a Friday evening. Gertie met us at the door.

"Come on in ladies. Alice, Clara great to see you both! It has been a long time."

"Thanks Gertie" I said. "Yes, it has. Tonight, Maw here will be my assistant. It's rather...peaceful for a Friday evening."

She sadly responded, "Yes, there was a tragedy in town. The steelworkers, which included most of my customers, were protesting. The governor sent in the National Guard, and the state militia. They had fired on the protesters. Seven men were killed. I knew a couple of them. The funeral was this afternoon."

I answered, "What a shame."

"Yes. But life goes on, doesn't it? We have a lady upstairs ready to bear a child. Her name is Bella. She has been working until last week. She claimed this birth is early, but I think she is quite large," replied Gertie. "Go on upstairs to the back room. When you get there, send down Bet. I need her help."

"Will do," I said.

I took Maw up the stairs, through the kitchen, to the stairway behind the pantry. The moans got louder as we walked down the hall.

I opened the door. The woman who must have been Bella laid on a bed. She looked like a woman who was close to giving birth. Her hair was a bit thrashed, and she was looking a bit exhausted.

"Hello Bella," I said. "We are both midwives, and we are here to care for you. My name is Alice, and this is my mother, Clara."

"Glad you made it."

I looked over at the lady assisting her, who must have been Bet. "Hello Bet — Gertie needs your help downstairs. Come back if you can."

I then asked, "Maw, could you set up the room while I get to know Bella better?"

"Sure Alice. Can do," replied Maw.

I sat next to Bella. "Tell me about your situation."

"I can between contractions. Oh, here comes another one — *whew, whew, whew!*" cried out Bella.

"This is my second pregnancy," she said. "My first one ended a lot sooner than this. And the baby did not survive. I got pretty big with this pregnancy, yet I feel this is early. I have had lots of nausea with this one. Baby is quite active. I am contemplating on keeping this baby. I have been talking with ladies at a local church who have members who will support me. They even have a room set up for me to stay in."

Soon, the labor pains were coming more frequent and much stronger.

"*Whew, whew, whew.* I can't take it. This is too much. *Whew, whew, whew.*"

"Breath with me, Bella. In through the nose, out through the mouth. Breath for your baby. You can do it."

"Okay. Okay. I can. I can." As Bella started deep breathing, her pains seemed to lessen.

I gazed around the room. I noticed it was a bit cleaner than most rooms I have used here at Gertie's place. I even saw a few baby blankets hanging on a chair. The linens were very clean.

"That sounds wonderful. Bella, you look comfortable — do you want to have your baby on this bed?" I asked.

Bella nodded. "Yes. I would hate to move at this time."

"Maw," I called. "Let's just move the waxed newspapers under her bottom. And let's grab that extra pail and keep it close to the end of the bed. It can catch any waste."

Within an hour, Bella was ready. Her contractions subsided, and she was able to gather strength as she got ready to birth. We helped her get comfortable.

Bella laid on her left side and threw her right leg up and over the bed to dangle, as this seemed to make her comfortable.

She attempted a few pushes then decided to sit up with both of her legs dangling off the bed. She was in sync as she took in a few deep breaths before she started to push.

I remarked, "Bella, you are really an expert with breathing. You look like a woman with experience."

Bella took deep full breaths between phrases. "When I was a kid —I assisted my mother with a few births. She was also a midwife. Sadly, she was tragically killed in a buggy accident when I was twelve." She got a worried look on her face. "Here comes a big one!"

Bella, Maw, and I started to breathe together; she rolled back on the bed, and we placed in her in a semi-sitting position.

"Here comes the baby," I said, as I placed gentle pressure just below her pubic bone. As the baby expelled, it made a corkscrew turn.

I handed Maw the baby so she could tend to her. The baby was mostly blue and only made a small grimace and gasping sounds as she struggled to breathe. Maw vigorously rubbed her back as she dried her off, while encouraging her to take in her first breath. The baby girl was completely covered with white cheese film, with fine hairs across her back and shoulders. She was quite small, and her head was quite big in relationship to its body.[B-25] This was quite a surprise, since Bella's abdomen was so large.

Within minutes, Maw was able to stimulate the baby to breathe. The first thing we witnessed was that the baby was pinking up. We heard a loud cry and the crackling lung sounds disappeared. Complete elation filled the room. I saw Bella smile. We all embraced the beautiful sound of a crying baby.

I announced, "It's a girl!"

Maw placed the baby on Bella's chest. Tears of joy filled Bella's eyes. "I will call her Linda, which means beautiful. It was my mother's name."

After the cord stopped pulsating, she tied it off on two sides close to the baby's belly and gave it a cut. Then the normal gush of blood came out as the cord lengthened. We knew, very soon, the placenta would follow.

We waited for nearly an hour. Finally, the placenta did expel, and I handed it to Maw. Then she placed it in a bowl.

At the same time, I was getting ready to massage the uterus down, when to my surprise I saw a loop of another blue cord come out.[B-26]

"What do we have here?" I asked. "Come here Maw look at this."

Maw immediately stepped in. "Bella, let me take Linda and place her in the bassinet." She swaddled the baby.

"Oh no! Is everything okay?" cried Bella.

I said, "Bella you are good. You are doing great. Listen to me. Let's turn you around and place your head on this pillow with your bottom up." Once she was on all fours, I let her know:

"Bella, you are having another baby."

Bella rolled her eyes.

Maw directed me. "Alice — just put gentle pressure to push the baby away from the cord. If possible."

I said, "Bella, I know it is hard to be in that position with your head down and bottom in the air. But we are going to have you blow instead of push for the first three rounds. Then, we will position as you desire."

We are doing this because when you push, we want your body to be extra ready."

Minutes later, the second baby started coming. Bella cried out.

"Ladies, it's coming! I can't stop."

"Maw, first grab the towel over there and inspect the baby, before placing her on Bella's chest."

"That's my plan, Alice!"

I said, "Here it comes!"

Quickly, the second baby came. It was another little girl.

I immediately handed her over to Maw. I noticed right away she was even smaller than the first baby. She was completely blue and quite floppy, with white cheesy material covering her body — and covered with fine hairs, especially on her shoulders.[B-25]

I could hear Maw whispering to the baby. "Breathe little one. Just take one breath. You can do it; I know you can," she murmured, as she forcefully rubbed the baby's back.

I saw Maw grab a corner of the towel and remove goo out of the baby's mouth. It didn't appear to help.

Maw kept working on stimulating the baby, as the placenta came out. It was small, and the cord was white, thin, and not sending blood to the baby.

Maw gave me a despondent look as she sadly shook her head. No words were said.

I knew just then that the baby had died.

Maw wrapped the baby and placed her in a box next to the sink. She was careful to wrap a fresh new blanket around her.

Meanwhile, Bella was becoming weak.

I massaged her belly right away. At first it seemed to work as I applied gentle pressure to the uterus, but then I noticed the uterus getting boggy. The bright red bleeding started to increase. I saw a few blood clots. To my dismay, the flood began.[B-10] Bella started breathing a bit faster as blood gushed out.

Immediately, I asked "Maw, how do those placentas look?"

"Let me see. The first one looks great, but the second one is missing a few chunks."[B-27]

"Okay, let me reach in and see if I can remove any placenta parts ... Yep, here are a few fragments ... Oh my, here it is a big chunk.[B-27] Maw stay with her; let me get some ergot. Let's first elevate her legs, she looks a bit clammy and pale."

I grabbed the ergot from my bag, and poured one dram into a wine cup sitting next to the bed, "Bella, could you sip on this?"

She could barely sip as I raised her head.

Finally, I was able to feel the uterus firming up. I applied direct pressure. Within ten minutes the bleeding subsided. We made it a priority to keep a close eye on Bella's bleeding and checked her uterus's firmness.

We attempted to give Bella lots of water to drink. She only took a few sips.

Bella softly announced, "I will call this little one Helen. As she is a light to us all showing us how precious life is."

Oh no, did she not realize her baby died?

I gave her time.

"Bella ... Maw, and I are so happy to see that you and your little baby Linda are doing better. We were quite worried for both of you." I found myself tearing up as I told her, "As for your second baby, I regret to tell you that she died."

"I know... but I can still call her Helen." Bella's eyes were full of tears.

"Of course, you can."

We could hear commotion outside the door. It was Bella's closest friends and co-workers from the house. Maw went outside to tell them about the two births. They were both saddened to hear about Helen — but relieved that Bella and Linda were fine.

Bella's friends came into the room and were in awe of the sweet baby Linda.

They gathered around Bella. Each one of them gave her hug. I thought this was a good time to show them how to care for Bella. I addressed them. "As you can see, Bella is a bit weak. She bled more than expected. Are you able to take turns caring for her in the night?"

They all nodded yes; I could tell they all loved Bella.

"Here is a chamber pot she can use to go to the bathroom in her bed. Don't let her walk until she can drink this whole pitcher of water and quits feeling dizzy. Please also encourage her to eat if she is hungry."

They all nodded their heads in agreement.

"Are any of you familiar with breastfeeding?"

To my surprise, they all raised their hands.

"You will see that her uterus cramps as she feeds her baby; we all know this can help to decrease the bleeding," I told them.

I then went on to show how to massage her belly and I even left some ergot for them to administer. I also left them an eyedropper in case the baby had trouble sucking.

Soon after we cleaned up the room, Maw and I left. Before we did, we walked over and gave Bella a great big hug.

I leaned over and told the baby, "Little Linda, you are lucky to have a mama that loves you so much. Live a good life."

We walked downstairs and said goodbye to Gertie. She handed us an envelope.

Maw said, "Hope to see you again. I love how you cleaned up this place."

We walked out and there was Albert waiting for us. We were so fortunate to have him.

"Ladies, may I help you into the buggy?"

We had a lovely long ride home. Maw complimented my work as a midwife, "Alice, without a doubt, you are a midwife. You are not the little girl birthing assistant I used to know. You handled this birth perfectly, and kept your composure and mind open, so you could make effective decisions. All while showing compassion as you cared for this woman and her babies."

"Thank you, Maw. You know I learned from the best! I not only feel like a midwife. I am a midwife!"

"Alice, what does a midwife mean to you?"

"A midwife means *"with woman."* Not only during good times, but also during difficult times of despair and sometimes remorse. This is especially important during a woman's time of pregnancy or giving birth."

"Okay then, what does birthing mean to you?"

"One of the greatest joys in life can be during the time you give birth, which can also be quite painful. It's truly a miracle to witness the creation a new life. As a young woman, having a period can be uncomfortable and even repulsive at times, but it helps build strength. This strength can be invaluable not only in childbirth and raising children, but also during difficult times as you navigate through life's unpredictable journey."

The buggy ride became bumpy as Albert pulled on the road next to the river.

"Maw, I finally know why you and Grandma had a 'could be' attitude."

"Really? What are your thoughts?"

"My hunting experience with Pa helped me gain perspective and understand that birthing is a unique experience that doesn't always rely on good skills for good outcomes. Even with a map filled with cues, I might still end up on the wrong road. The human body is complex, and there is still so much we don't fully understand. However, your 'could be' attitude made me consider alternative complications that could present and have helped me maintain an open mind and remain vigilant for new cues."

"Alice, I have been meaning to ask you. What have you decided about nursing school?"

"I am not going, Maw. Not at this time. I realize I definitely want to stay with midwifing ... and I do love Josef. But not sure where that will go."

Maw seemed disappointed. "You could always change your mind."

I smiled at her. "Could be."

All I did know, is that when I got home, I needed to restock my birthing bag as I get ready for the next birth.

Susan E. Fleming

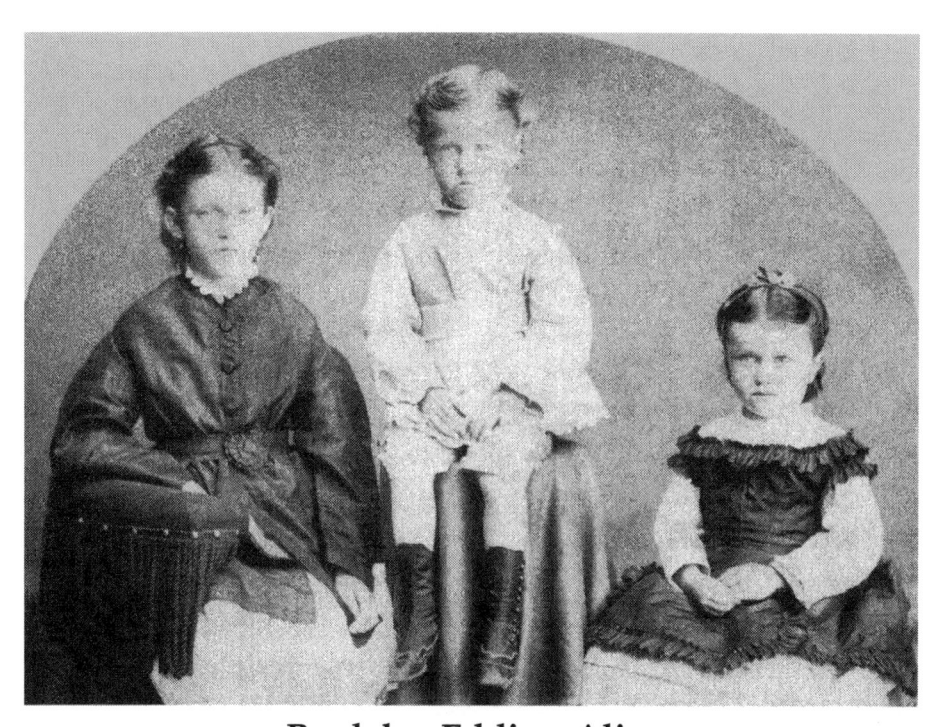

**Beulah – Eddie – Alice
1874 Madison Wisconsin**

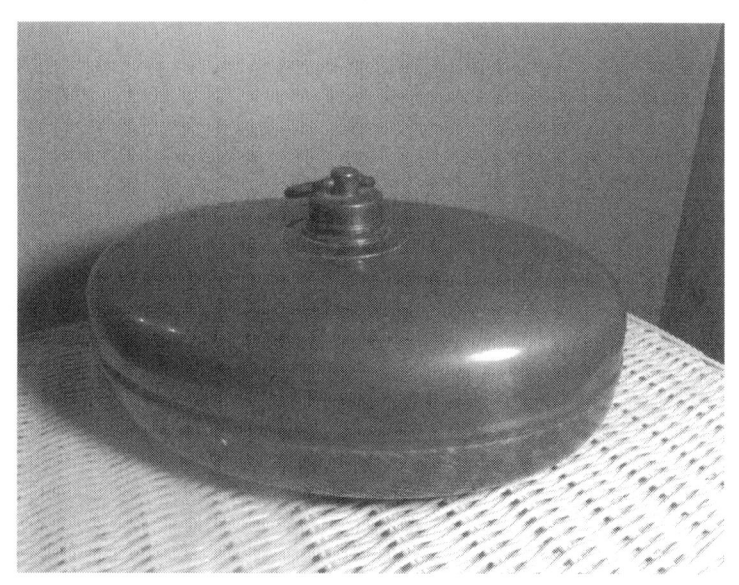

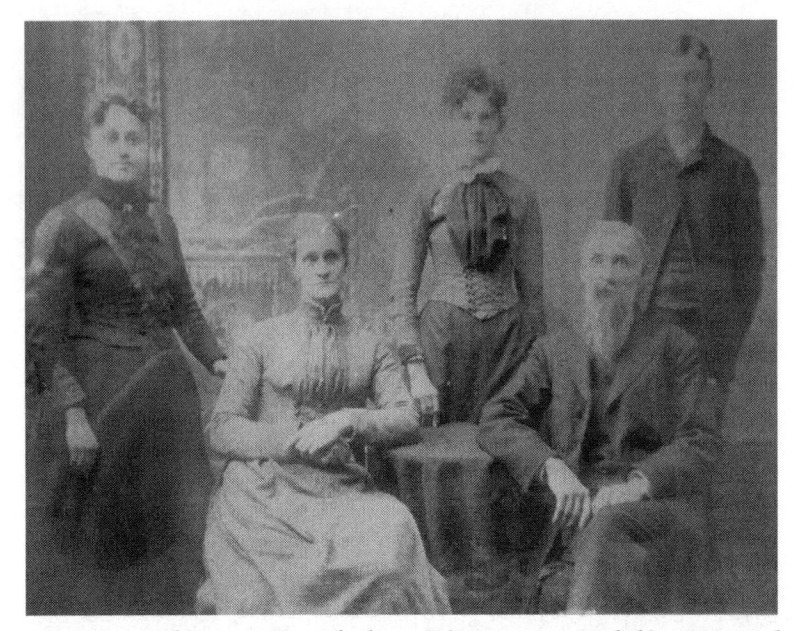

Alice – Clara – Beulah – Pierson - Eddie Wood
Milwaukee Wisconsin
1886

Birthing - Current Basic Definitions and Explanations

*Please see a birthing practitioner for more detailed information regarding the following. B1 to B27

1. **Move the Mom — Move the Baby.** *Freedom of movement is important in making the birth of your baby easier. It is the best way to use gravity to help your baby come down and increase the size and shape of your pelvis. It allows you to respond to pain in an active way, and it may speed up the labor process* (Simkin & Ancheta, 2005). *"Squatting increases the size of the pelvic outlet."* Dr. Katherine Camacho Carr CNM

2. **Uterine Massage.** Uterine massage following the expulsion of the placenta is a component of the active management of routine labor recommended by the International Confederation of Midwives (ICM) and International Federation of Gynecology and Obstetrics (FIGO). However, the precise benefit is still undetermined. Pg 1036 Varney's. Anecdotal stories from Midwives in European countries often take a gentler approach. At times, only when massaging is indicated. Alice gently massaged the fundus (top of the uterus); then held constant pressure on the firm uterus for two minutes following the routine births. **AVOID VIGOROUS MASSAGE** on routine births, which can increase bleeding. This was a story the author heard from an Icelandic Midwife working in Texas.

3. **Milia:** White dots on the nose of the newborn. Common occurrences will resolve on their own. Do not squeeze. Pg 1214 Varney's

4. **Bring the baby down to the ground, then up to the sky.** The author has heard OB-GYNs and Midwives describe assisting a woman during the actual birth.

5. **Secret Salve.** This story of Clara and Pierson was told to the author by her Grandmother, Marie. Alice's youngest daughter.

6. **Short Cords.** Personal experience of the author, who noticed that when the cord is short or there is tension on the cord. That she noticed extra bleeding during the birth.

7. **Breech Birth:** When a fetus presents during birth with buttocks or feet. This can be a serious condition as the baby is birthed. Leaving the large head to birth last and possibly stopping blood flow to the umbilical cord. Incidence 3% to 4 % of Births at term. It is important to see a birthing provider who is skilled with breech births. Pg. 1006 *Varney's*

8. **Rick Brazell's Hunting account.** Avid hunter and founder of the First Hunt Foundation gave his approval and suggestions for Alice's first hunt with her father.

9. **Professor Hollins Martin** gave this account of her cameo appearance in the book: When I arrived at the tale of Miss Caroline Hollinsworth (page 141 - 150), I smiled and thought, "What a synchronicity". Caroline Hollinsworth in 1875 was certified as a nurse at the City of Edinburgh's General Lying-In Hospital and progressed to become a midwifery tutor. With similarity, my name in Caroline Hollins Martin and I was born in Edinburgh in 1962 and have spent the last 10 years of my 40-year career as a midwife who teaches students their craft.

10. **Post-Partum Hemorrhage:** Is considered Early if it occurs in the first 24 hours. Or late if it occurs from 24 hours to 6 weeks postpartum. Incidence is 2% to 3 % of all births. Most literature defines PPH as a blood loss of 500 ml to 1000 ml depending on the type of birth. Pg 1044. *Varney's*

11. **Placenta Previa:** is defined as when the placenta implants over the inner cervical os or opening. The bright red bleeding, as explained by Ms. Hollingsworth, is a current sign today. Incidence 0.4% of births. —pg 1001. *Varney's*

12. **Semmelweis Story.** In the mid-1880s, this story was disseminated throughout Europe and even during the Civil War. This led to hand washing.

13. **Placenta Abruption:** defined as a premature separation of a normally implanted placenta. The rigid Abdomen and dark blood, [old blood] that Alice saw are current signs today. The kick to the abdomen, such as with Emma, or following off a buggy could

cause the placenta to abrupt. Incidence 1% of births. — pg 1001. *Varney's*.

14. **Clara Civil War Story**. Part of the family history of the author's great-great-grandmother

15. **RH Factor** (Inherited): Rh negative women do not have the RH factor protein attached to their blood cells, but if they are exposed to an Rh positive baby, they can create antibodies that will attack the second Rh positive baby in an attempt to destroy it, which can lead to serious health problems including death for the baby. Rhogam was developed in the late 1960s as a means to treat this. Today we consider Rhogam a *Forgotten Miracle*. — pg 674 — *Varney's*

16. **Tearing from the Urethra with Hands-Free Birthing**. This is an opinion of Alice based on her and the author's experiences. *"Tearing near the urethra (periurethral tears) are usually caused by a deflexed head and/or rapid delivery of the head. That's why we place our hands on the head — to keep it flexed presenting the smallest diameter of the head to the perineum and prevention of torpedoes!"* Dr. Katherine Camacho Carr CNM

17. **Chewing Chalk**. There was a history of recommending chalk for indigestion in the 1880s. Please see your provider for updated treatments.

18. **Preeclampsia:** Many theories describe preeclampsia, including having a new partner as what happened with Emma. The most common definition is related to hypertension, urinary protein, liver, and renal assessment. Edema of the face, hands and visual disturbances and headaches may occur. Incidence is 6% to 10% of woman experience hypertension during pregnancy. Pg 745 — 747 *Varney's*

19. **HELLP Syndrome** is an acronym for hypertension, elevated liver enzymes, and low platelets. It can be a dangerous sequela of preeclampsia or a separate disorder. Up to 20% of women with HELLP do not have hypertension. A severe headache with visual disturbances, upper middle of the abdomen

(epigastric) pain, and yellowing of the skin (jaundice) that Emma was experiencing can indicate severe preeclampsia or HELLP Syndrome, which are both life-threatening and could lead to DIC. Pg 747 *Varney's*

20. **Fetal Demise.** A blue baby is indicative of recent oxygen deprivation. Emma's baby was white, which indicates longer oxygen deprivation. Initially the baby is warm but quickly becomes cool to the touch. You may see the lips being dark purple, which turns black. This is based on the author's experiences of caring for babies who died in utero.

21. **Eclampsia - Seizures:** Seizures were known as Fits in the 1800s. If seizures occur in a woman with preeclampsia and no other cause, it is considered eclampsia. Pg 746 *Varney's*

22. **Disseminated intravascular coagulation [DIC]:** DIC results in the depletion of platelets and results in uncontrolled bleeding. This was seen in Emma as she was dying. Pg 1044 Varney's

23. **Gestational Diabetes** Historically, used to describe diabetes that is first noticed during pregnancy. Most likely the Becker Sisters had type two related to their dietary intake. Pg 740 Varney

24. **Shoulder Dystocia:** Impaction of the anterior shoulder behind the pubic Bone. Impaction of the posterior shoulder on the sacral promontory. This results in **turtling,** which the head emerges and retracts during the pushing phase of the birth. According to the story, Alice, Clara, and Grandma knew they witnessed turtling with large women who were birthing. Rolling a Mom on all four is considered the 4th maneuver; in this story, it was the go-to or when all else fails method. Pg 1016 *Varney's*

25. **Premature Newborn:** The head appears larger in comparison to the baby's body. **Vernix-** White cheesy substance of dead cells and sebaceous secretions. Increases with gestational age. Protects the newborn in utero. **Lanugo** — fine downy hair on shoulders — back. Decreases with gestational age. Pg 112 — 1214. Varney's

26. **Overt Prolapsed Cord:** defined as the umbilical cord completely slips out of the cervix and is protruding the vagina prior to the baby being birthed. An obstetric emergency. Often requiring an emergency cesarean surgery. Pg 1021 *Varney's*

27. **Retained Placenta:** The World Health Organization defines retained placenta as longer than 30 minutes but recommends waiting another 30 minutes before manually removing it unless hemorrhaging is present. Incidence 0.01% to 6.3 % of births. pg 1042 Varney's

28. **The Emma and Uri story.** Is based on the author's grandfather's stories. William Harrison McMillen. Grandpa Harry's own father left his mother with two children under three years of age in the mountain town of Silverton, Colorado in the 1890s. Soon after, his mother married a Jewish man in town who owned a hat store. Many years later, after Harry returned from WWI in 1919 he married the love of his life and one year later his wife died in his arms at 7 months pregnant. The family story was that she had kidney failure.

King, T. L., Brucker, M. C., Kriebs, J. M.,Fahey, J. O. (2013, October 21). *Varney's Midwifery*. Jones & Bartlett Learning.

Playfair, W.S. (1880). *Playfair's System of Midwifery*. 3rd edition.{American Edition} Philadelphia: Henry C. Lea.

Simkin P, Ancheta R. 2005. *The labor progress handbook* (2nd ed.) Malden, MA: Blackwell Science

Healthcare in America during the 1880s — Education - Infections - Septic Shock:

In the 1880s, American healthcare education was truly in its infancy, including in Wisconsin. Medical, midwifery, and nursing schools were non-existent for most Americans traveling west. By 1870, there were only three nursing schools in the United States. Mostly in the Northeast. Unlike in Europe, medical school certificates were easy to obtain after a six-week course.

Back in 1880 America, people were aware of illnesses such as smallpox, typhoid fever, and venereal diseases, but they didn't have a clear understanding of infections. Even though the Semmel Weiss story was useful, it was challenging to spread the word among the general public and healthcare providers. They did know that keeping food clean and washed could prevent spoilage, and many thought the same could hold for their bodies.

In the early 1860s, the Civil War taught many lessons, but unfortunately, many people suffered, such as when numerous legs were amputated without considering the risk of infection. However, doctors and nurses worked tirelessly to save lives.

H1 - Special thanks to the following websites, which enriched the stories being told in this book:
University of Wisconsin — Encyclopedia of Milwaukee
https://emke.uwm.edu/entry/workers-movements/
Milwaukee PBS — The Making of Milwaukee
https://www.milwaukeepbs.org/the-making-of-milwaukee/history/
Milwaukee Historical Society https://milwaukeehistory.net/
American Battlefield Trust https://www.battlefields.org/learn/articles/brief-overview-american-civil-war

H-2 Playfair, W.S. (1880). *Playfair's System of Midwifery*. 3rd edition. {American Edition} Philadelphia: Henry C. Lea.

H-3 Morten, H, (1900.) *The Midwives Pocket Book*. London: The Scientific Press, Limited.

UPCOMING RELEASES

The prequel to this book is coming soon (estimated Fall 2024), featuring the early life of Clara French Wood 1850s – 1870s.

New York Frontier Midwife – Nurse: Clara French
A Civil War Story

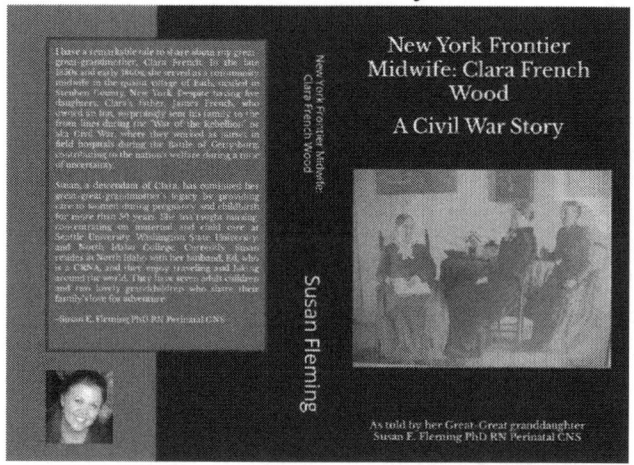

The sequel to this book will be coming in Fall 2025:

South Dakota Midwife: Alice Ada Wood
Deadwood SD

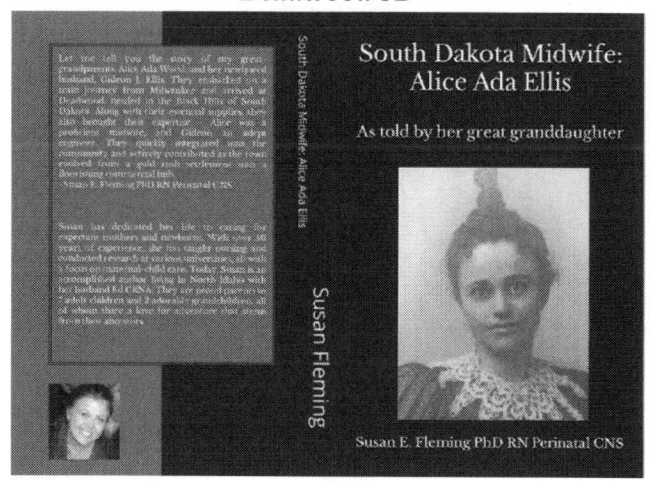

ORIGINAL BOOK

The original sequel to all of these books. Originally published in 2013. 4th Edition published June 2023

**Seattle Pioneer Midwife: Alice Ada Wood Ellis
Midwife, Nurse & Mother to All**

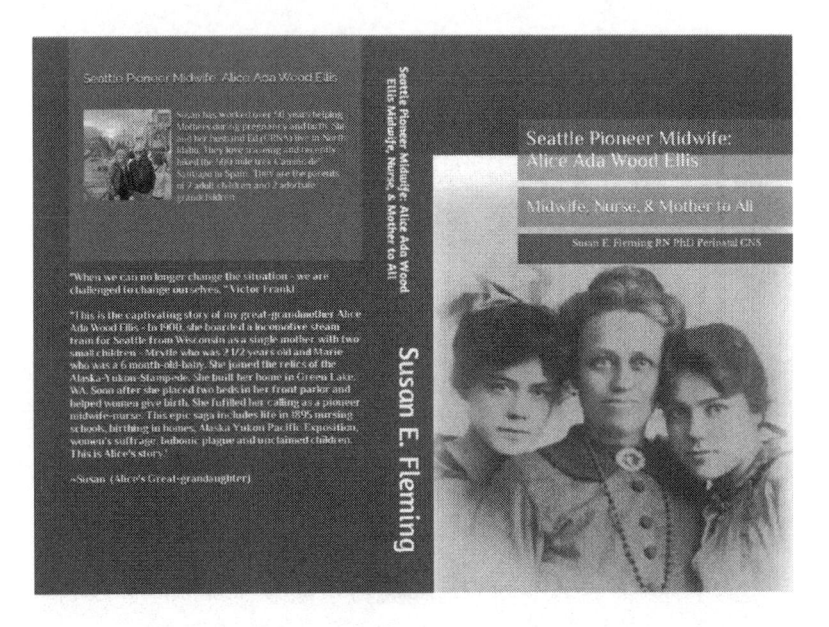

You can find these books in libraries and local bookstores as well

as Amazon.

Printed in Great Britain
by Amazon